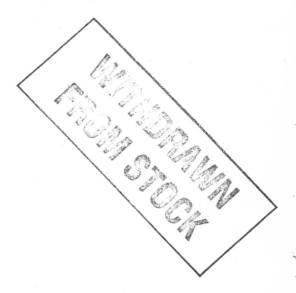

Isolated Organ Perfusion

Isolated Organ Perfusion

Edited by

H. D. RITCHIE
Professor of Surgery, London Hospital Medical College

and

J. D. HARDCASTLE
Professor of Surgery, Nottingham University

Crosby Lockwood Staples   London

Granada Publishing Limited
First published in Great Britain 1973 by Crosby Lockwood Staples
Park Street St Albans and 3 Upper James Street London W1R 4BP

ISBN 0 258 96890 7
Printed in Great Britain by
C Tinling & Co Ltd
London and Prescot

Contributors

H. D. Ritchie   *Professor of Surgery, The London Hospital*

J. D. Hardcastle   *Professor of Surgery, The University of Nottingham*

W. E. R. Green   *Lecturer in Surgery, The London Hospital*

R. J. Nicholls   *Lecturer in Surgery, The London Hospital*

P. A. Thomas   *Wellcome Surgical Research Fellow*

B. R. Simpson   *Professor of Anaesthesia, The London Hospital*

L. Strunin   *Assistant Director, Anaesthetic Unit, The London Hospital*

J. Hermon-Taylor   *Reader in Surgery, The London Hospital*

A. D. W. Maclean   *Assistant Director, Surgical Unit, The London Hospital*

R. D. Cohen   *Reader in Medicine, The London Hospital*

J. M. Beaugié   *Senior Surgical Registrar, The London Hospital*

R. A. Iles   *Research Assistant, The London Hospital*

Margaret H. Lloyd   *Research Assistant, The London Hospital*

Contents

Contributors   v

Acknowledgements   viii

1 Introduction   1
   H. D. Ritchie

Part One

2 Basic Requirements and Principles   9
   H. D. Ritchie
   J. D. Hardcastle
3 Choice of Animal   16
   H. D. Ritchie
4 Anaesthesia   20
   B. R. Simpson
   L. Strunin
5 Apparatus   30
   W. E. R. Green
6 Perfusion Fluid and Choice of Flow Rate   52
   R. J. Nicholls
7 Monitoring   60
   P. A. Thomas

Part Two

8 **Liver**

Dog   71
R. J. Nicholls
Anaesthesia and the Isolated Liver   100
B. R. Simpson
L. Strunin
Pig   111
J. M. Beaugié
Rat   120
R. D. Cohen
R. A. Iles
M. H. Lloyd

9 **Stomach**

Basic Preparation   135
W. E. R. Green
P. A. Thomas
Assessment of Preparation   150
W. E. R. Green
P. A. Thomas

10 **Duodenum and Pancreas**

Basic Preparation   171
J. Hermon-Taylor
Gallbladder and Bile Ducts   191
A. D. W. Maclean

Index   209

Acknowledgements

We wish to acknowledge help from the following:

Miss R. Auden	Xenon studies
Mr P. Knight	Technical
Mr M. Hutton	
Miss D. Tolfree	
Miss J. Bungener	Secretarial
Miss P. Gillam	
Miss L. Pepall	

Most of the work described in this volume was made possible by the generosity of the Board of Governors of The London Hospital and the authors concerned wish to record their gratitude to them for providing the facilities and the financial support which made it possible.

Mr Roger Green and Mr John Nicholls did part of this work during tenure of M.R.C. awards.

Mr Paul Thomas received support from the Board of Governors of The London Hospital and from the Wellcome Trust.

CHAPTER ONE

Introduction

Organs have been isolated and perfused for several different purposes; sometimes in order to preserve them for subsequent transplantation; sometimes for therapeutic purposes as when cytotoxic drugs are circulated or in the treatment of liver failure; but classically to increase our knowledge of their physiology or patho-physiology. It is with the last of these that this book is concerned. In fact it aims to provide a general background of the scientific and technical knowledge which the research worker will need to embark on a project involving perfusion of a viscus. It will attempt to describe the technique of perfusion of several abdominal organs and to indicate the sort of measurements and studies which can be made on each.

Whilst the perfusion of isolated organs has been an established scientific method of studying visceral physiology since the classical studies of Dale in the early 1930s, little effort has been made to date to apply these techniques to the examination of problems more relevant to clinical work. Although in recent years, perfusion studies on the liver in shock (Hardcastle and Ritchie, 1968) and the effect of anaesthetic agent on the liver (Strunin et al, 1969) have shown that much can be learned from such an approach.

It is perhaps particularly appropriate at this time that there should be an increase in the volume of this type of study since the technological basis of organ perfusion has recently been so greatly improved by advances made in the field of whole-body perfusion.

Two further considerations seem worthy of mention. Firstly, to make these preparations, a fairly high standard of surgical skill is required from the young experimentalist, be he physiologist, pharmacologist or surgeon. Nevertheless it is clear to us from an experience of some 1,500 isolated organ perfusion experiments that where the laboratory is attuned to such studies and the technical help and guidance good enough, workers new to research can embark with confidence on a project using isolated perfused organs.

Secondly, organ perfusion studies offer a half-way house between studies on the whole animal and *in vitro* experiments. Such studies are of the acute variety and may be feasible where time or animal accommodation is limited.

But it is not from such conveniences that the chief scientific value of organ perfusion studies arises. Rather it is from the precision and specificity of the responses which can be observed. For example, when gastrin is given to an intact animal it can be shown that bile flow is markedly increased, but few conclusions can be drawn about the mechanism of this response from such a study. Gastrin stimulates acid secretion – acid in the duodenum promotes secretin release – secretin is a potent stimulant of bile flow. Hence it is difficult to tell in the intact animal whether this is the mechanism which is operating or whether, for example, gastrin itself is acting directly on the liver without secretin as the intermediary. Only in the perfused preparation can it be demonstrated whether or not the substance being studied has a direct effect on the viscus.

The other major advantage of the perfused preparation is that its blood flow, gaseous exchange and temperature are under direct continuous control. This enables quantitative studies of the effect of deliberately induced changes in these parameters to be made. For example, the effects of reduced blood flow, anoxia, hypothermia, changes in blood pH or osmolarity can be established, the results of nerve stimulation assessed or the electrical and motor activity in a viscus recorded under relatively stable controlled conditions. Such studies, however, can only be meaningful if the function of the organ has not been adversely affected by the isolation and perfusion.

Feasibility

Many organs have already been successfully perfused. Amongst these are the liver, kidney, spleen, lung, heart, pancreas, stomach, duodenum, biliary tree, small bowel with ileo-caecal junction, colon, adrenal gland, bone, uterus and ovary. Some of these present peculiar difficulties of their own such as the liver which tends to develop hepatic venous spasm or the kidney which may develop arterial spasm or the lung which is prone to become oedematous. But our experience shows that, with thoughtfulness and effort, these problems are capable of solution in the light of the present-day knowledge of perfusion technology. Whilst, therefore, there are general principles which may guide us in any perfusion undertaking, one has constantly to be on the look-out for idiosyncrasies in the organ itself since only thus may the best results be obtained. Species vary of course and a viscus in one species may more readily lend itself to perfusion than its anatomical counterpart in another.

What is not possible at present is to achieve prolonged perfusions which would permit the study of visceral function over several days. Most of the preparations we describe here will behave in a reasonably physiological way, as far as we can establish this by testing, for up to four or five hours. Clearly, therefore, most phenomena which can be studied in such a preparation are of the acute variety. It is, however, possible to finesse this difficulty in various ways. For example, one can produce biliary obstruction by tying the common bile duct in an animal several days before perfusion is carried out. In this way one can get nearer to what is happening in the liver at this stage of the process even if one cannot yet follow it along *ab initio*.

Extensions

What of the future? We have already achieved perfusions of combinations of organs simultaneously. This has advantages in that it may pin-point an interaction between the two or allow for the study of more complex combined functions. We shall see below how the duodenum, pancreas, stomach and biliary tree may be included in one preparation. We have perfused stomach and oesophagus and also stomach and liver together. Such preparations may offer exciting new possibilities for the future. They are technically within our grasp at the present.

But it is not only in the multiplicity of the viscera involved that the field of organ perfusion will be extended. It is now possible to measure the tissue spaces and compartments in the single viscus in much the same way as hitherto whole-body studies have been carried out in man. We shall see below that inulin space, tritiated water space and other parameters such as red cell mass and albumin pool can be measured simultaneously in the liver. This is also at a time when bile, liver lymph and blood entering and leaving the liver can be sampled, the liver meanwhile being weighed continuously throughout the study. This degree of resolution may be expected to give a much clearer picture of the intrahepatic scene under a variety of circumstances than has been available hitherto.

Much will be added to the scope of perfusion studies when prolonged experiments can be carried out. We shall see below that oedema in the viscus seems to be the main limiting factor in extending the duration of perfusion with present techniques. It seems likely that oxygenators and pumps which cause less trauma to the blood are a major prerequisite for this. Much work is going on in this field at present and we shall describe our experience of membrane oxygenators in this context. It must be recognised, however, that at present this is a significant limitation in the method. When prolonged perfusion becomes feasible more advanced studies, for example on absorption, metabolism, elaboration of proteins, degradation of toxic substances, etc., will bring us much new information. It is however in the study of developing infective disease and perhaps even neoplasia during extended perfusion experiments that the greatest future interest may lie.

Its place as a technique for studying basic visceral function in the gastro-intestinal, renal and cardiovascular field would seem already to be assured. What then of neural tissue? Cerebral perfusion is certainly feasible. As a group we have only a small experience of this from cytotoxicity studies on the canine subject. Clearly, neurophysiological phenomena might with profit be examined in this way and also the effect of stereotactic procedures on these. The barriers to this sort of work are not likely to be technical.

In general terms therefore we can say that perfusion studies on isolated organs have much to offer. They provide an excellent basic training in setting up anatomically complex preparations, in multiple sophisticated monitoring techniques and an almost limitless opportunity to examine intrinsic visceral function. They can be used in the grand physiological manner to elicit basic responses (Andrews et al, 1953), more intimately to study at the cellular level metabolic processes freed from the effects of extrinsic neural or hormonal stimuli (Cohen et al, 1971, Iles et al, 1972) or even to examine the local effects of pathologic processes or surgical procedures on a viscus. (See below "Anaesthesia and the Isolated Liver".)

We cannot hope to cover authoritatively all existing perfusion techniques in this volume. Rather we have chosen to describe in detail those with which we have most familiarity. The preparations to be described are therefore exclusively gastro-intestinal but much basic perfusion lore, valid we believe for such studies on any viscus, will be offered in the hope that our experience in this fascinating field may be of use to others.

References

Andrews, W.H.H., Hecker, R., Maegraith, B.G. and Ritchie, H.D. (1953) Direct connections between hepatic artery and hepatic veins in the canine liver. *J. Physiol.* **122** *Proc. Physiol. Soc.* 24–25 July.

Andrews, W.H.H., Hecker, R., Maegraith, B.G. and Ritchie, H.D. (1953) Constriction within the canine hepatic venous tree. *J. Physiol.* **122,** *Proc. Physiol. Soc.* 24–25 July.

Bauer, W., Dale, H.H., Poulsson, L.T. and Richards, D.W. (1932) The control of circulation through the liver. *J. Physiol.* **74,** 343.

Cohen, R.D., Iles, R.A., Barnett, D., Howell, M.E.O. and Strunin, J.M. (1971) The effect of changes in lactate uptake on the intracellular pH of the perfused rat liver. *Clinical Science* **41,** 159.

Hardcastle, J.D., and Ritchie, H.D. (1968) The liver in shock. *Brit. J. Surg.* **54,** 679.

Iles, R.A., Barnett, D., Strunin, L., Strunin, J.M., Simpson, B.R. and Cohen, R.D. (1972) The effect of hypoxia on succinate metabolism in man and the isolated perfused dog liver. *Clinical Science* **42,** 35.

Strunin, L., Coultas, R.J., Walker, W.D., Strunin, J.M., Reynard, A. and Simpson, B.R. (1969) A comparison of the effects of halothane and methoxyflurane in the isolated perfused canine liver. *Brit. J. Anaesthesia* **41,** 790.

PART ONE

CHAPTER TWO

Basic Requirements and Principles

It must be recognised in all organ perfusion experiments that one is dealing with an isolated perfused denervated viscus usually from an animal. There is, therefore, no means by which results obtained in such experiments can immediately be taken to show what happens in man. We hope however in this volume to illustrate the sort of information which can be derived and must leave it to the reader to judge for himself the potential and relevance of such work.

Inevitably in a huge field such as whole-body perfusion and in the smaller one concerned with viscera, a jargon has grown up with which workers inexperienced in this sort of work may be unfamiliar. 'Priming volume' which means the minimum amount of perfusion fluid needed adequately to charge the whole system of tubes, pumps and oxygenator or 'cavitation' which refers to the distraction of the blood in the tubing leading to a pulsatile pump as it is sucked in during diastole are examples of terms which may lead to obscurities. An attempt will be made to explain such terms where they appear first of all in the text.

We find that certain basic principles are common to all the perfusion work we have done. The choice of animal, anaesthetic and operative technique, the apparatus and perfusion fluid and the monitoring and assessment of the preparation are technical factors of major importance and will be dealt with in some detail later in this section. Requiring less detailed description but vital to success are some less obvious procedural points.

Avoidance of Hypoxia

Of primary importance is the avoidance of hypoxia in the organ to be perfused. This can be achieved e.g., in the canine liver by allowing the animal to continue to pass blood into the hepatic artery whilst the portal vein is being cannulated; or in setting up stomach perfusion using a segment of aorta so that the animal supplies blood from the proximal end, whilst the distal end is cannulated. Most perfused organs react badly to hypoxia at this or any stage. In the liver, for example, within thirty seconds of the oxygenator being excluded from the circuit, potassium is lost from the cells and high levels appear in the venous blood (Figure 1). Recovery may be possible when the hypoxic damage is limited, but the time taken for this to occur may limit the usefulness of the experiment.

If isolation of the organ is impossible without temporary interruption of the arterial supply, the organ may be cooled so as to reduce the development of severe hypoxic changes. In the perfused liver cooling to 15°C completely prevents the changes induced during a short period of ischaemia at normal temperature (Hardcastle and Ritchie, 1968).

Hypoxia in the donor animal with the risk of catecholamine release and its associated nervous and vascular responses should be avoided. It was realised many years ago that once the 'blue' state in a liver (Andrews, Hecker, Maegraith and Ritchie, 1955) was developed, the preparation was not likely to recover and should be discarded.

Similarly trauma from handling the organ must be kept to a minimum. Oedema frequently results and in the case of gut, for example, the viscus behaves in an abnormal way thereafter.

Use of the Animal's Own Blood

Theoretically the ideal perfusion fluid is undiluted autologous blood. We have evidence that some livers respond by hepatic vein spasm when perfused with heterologous blood. The bowel seems less sensitive. For canine perfusion we have always found it possible to use autologous blood but dilution is sometimes necessary. This is in part due to the fact that it is not always possible to get an adequate priming volume from limited bleeding of the animal before starting to perfuse. If, of course, one bleeds the animal right out then large amounts of catecholamines and probably other metabolic and vaso-active substances may appear in the perfusate and the preparation suffers. There are other objections to whole blood relating to its

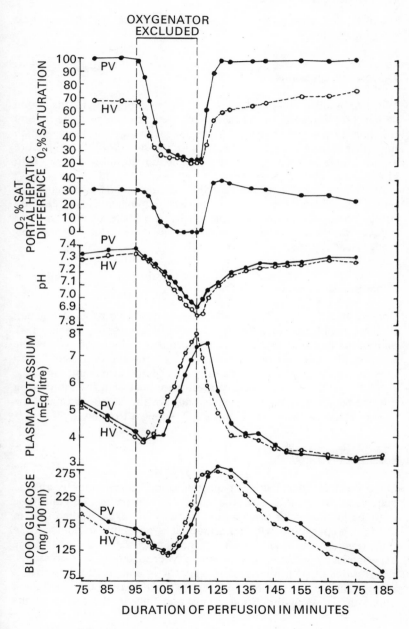

Fig. 1 *Effect of excluding the oxygenator during perfusion.*

viscosity and vulnerability in a perfusion circuit but these will be discussed below.

Disposable Apparatus

Where possible all apparatus which is in contact with the blood should be disposable. Although, as we shall see below in the section on apparatus, certain plastic tubings appear to lake substances which may have deleterious effects (Guess and Stetson, 1968). It is therefore an advantage to keep the amount of plastic material in contact with blood to a minimum.

Wide-bore tubes only increase the priming volume and hence are undesirable. This is particularly so where biochemical studies are being carried out since dilution of the substance being measured reduces the accuracy of measurement and may in certain circumstances lead to failure to detect it at all.

Experimental Team and their Duties

For the making of perfusion studies it is desirable to have a group of three people to constitute a team, each having his specific task allotted to him and familiar with the time at which his part in the experiment is to be played. We advise that there should be an operator, an assistant and an anaesthetist/pump attendant. Once the perfusion has begun any one of these may deal with the monitoring but one person should take responsibility for the venous drainage, the level of blood in the reservoir and the O_2 supply throughout.

Extent of Perfusion

Once the technique has been mastered and the operator is able to achieve perfusion it is wise to check the extent of this. Obviously he must be familiar with the relevant anatomy but even granted this, in the first preparations which are made it is advisable to demonstrate the extent of the tissue which has been perfused at the end of the experiment by injecting a solution of Micropaque at low pressures. Illustrations of such injections will appear in later sections. Suffice it to say that they offer a ready check on whether or not the perfusion apparatus is supplying blood evenly and fully to the tissues of the organ.

Experimental Procedure

Lastly in procedural considerations we must think of the plan of an experiment itself. Organs in general respond to the trauma of isolation and being set up for perfusion by exhibiting an initial period of 30–60 minutes during which they appear to be recovering from the manoeuvre. During this period in the liver e.g., potassium and glucose are lost, high levels being found in the hepatic venous blood (Figure 2). This change is reversed after about 30 minutes of adequate perfusion. It is important therefore in planning an experiment to allow this period to pass and to achieve the normal monitored parameters, described below in the section on the appropriate viscus, before beginning the test period. Otherwise much may be lost and the experiment invalidated.

This phenomenon of 'recovery' in such preparations is of considerable interest but has not been studied extensively. Presumably degrees of hypoxia and trauma contribute but sympathetic nervous stimulation and catecholamine release during the initial phases of the operation may be important factors.

In describing this period one is in reality referring to recovery from a transient period of deterioration in the preparation. Obviously with present techniques a final and irreversible state of deterioration will in due course ensue. As mentioned above, most of the canine preparations described here will be suitable for use for 4–5 hours but all gradually deteriorate and after that time most have become unreliable. In the liver for instance oedema gradually develops. This has been shown by weighing and histology. Accompanying this and perhaps preceding it is a slow continual rise in the portal venous pressure associated sometimes with a minor degree of outflow block. In the stomach oedema occurs, the mucosa becomes haemorrhagic and motor and electrical activity may become disorganised. It is essential to recognise these stigmata of deterioration in a preparation as they occur, since studies carried out under such circumstances are suspect.

Clearly damage to the blood in the perfusion circuit is also contributory. W.B.C.s and platelets are slowly destroyed and the residue of these may be identified in the tubing and on the plates or screens of the oxygenator as the experiment progresses. R.B.C.s are of course also damaged perhaps mainly by cavitation or grinding in the pumps. These should be tested to establish how much haemolysis they produce but not with an organ in the circuit since it will filter out much of the free haemoglobin and so give false low levels.

Essential metabolites such as glucose must be provided for the

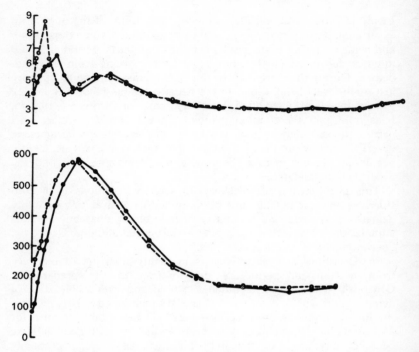

Fig. 2 Glucose and potassium levels in the portal and hepatic venous blood during isolated canine liver perfusion. The period during which measurements shown were made was th hours. Hepatic vein levels are shown by the dotted lines.

isolated organ. The degree to which this is required will depend on the nature and duration of the study.

If good preparations are to be made and meaningful data obtained we recommend strict adherence to these general principles. But what of the technical factors mentioned above as being specially important?

References

Andrews, W.H.H., Hecker, R., Maegraith, B.G., and Ritchie, H.D. (1955) The action of adrenaline, l-noradrenaline, acetyl choline and other substances on the blood vessels of the perfused canine liver. *J. Physiol.* **128,** 413.

Basic Requirements and Principles 15

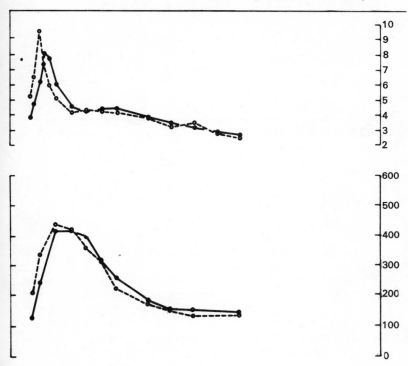

Guess, W.L., and Stetson, J.B. (1968) Tissue reactions to organotonin stabilised P.V.C. catheters *J. Am. Med. Ass.* **204,** 580.

Hardcastle, J.D., and Ritchie, H.D. (1968) The liver in shock. *Brit. J. Surg.* **55,** (5), 365A.

CHAPTER THREE

Choice of Animal

Various factors may determine choice and here the problem to be investigated will often be the determinant.

For studies on bile flow or composition for example, and in particular where large volumes of bile are required for analysis, the dog and the rabbit will be most suitable. The dog has the great advantage that it is not a herbivore and much of our knowledge of biliary physiology is based on canine work. Where, however, a metabolic or cellular phenomenon is to be studied the rat liver preparation may be perfectly adequate and is much more simple and economic to use.

Availability, cost, accommodation and dietary or species or other individual characteristics may be important considerations. Small animals are cheap, easy to house and readily available. The rat for example has been used most extensively (Miller *et al*, 1951; Brauer *et al*, 1951; Burton *et al*, 1960; Gunberg *et al*, 1955; Mortimer, 1961) and we include a chapter giving our experience with this technique. The rabbit (Andrews *et al*, 1956; Lundsgaard, 1938; Young *et al*, 1955; Price *et al*, 1957), the cat (Andrews *et al*, 1956; Lundsgaard, 1938; Corey and Britton, 1941), and the frog (Craig, 1958, 1959, 1963), have also been used. All have the disadvantage that they are small and have a small blood volume and small blood vessels. It is difficult to prime a perfusion circuit with autologous blood under such circumstances, so that donor blood or even asanguineous perfusion fluids may have to be used. To our way of thinking these are serious limitations in a preparation. But none the less much useful information on metabolic processes and the like has come from such studies.

With larger animals most of these problems can be overcome. If over 20 kg they usually have a blood volume large enough to 'prime' a perfusion circuit without so 'shocking' the animal in the process that the organ is seriously damaged before perfusion can be set up. The blood vessels of course are larger and more readily cannulated as are lymphatic trunks and main ducts such as the biliary or pancreatic duct. In the liver, for example, it is possible to perfuse both the hepatic artery and the portal vein, something which is technically very difficult in the rat, so that the preparations in theory at least have more claim to be physiological. It will become clear however, from what appears later in this book, that such experiments are more costly.

Amongst the larger animals which have been used are pig (Eiseman et al, 1961, 1963, 1964), calves (Chapman et al, 1960, 1961), sheep (Eiseman et al, 1961), goats (McCarthy et al, 1958), monkeys (Andrews et al, 1956) and of course the dog (Hardcastle and Ritchie, 1967, 1968; Hardcastle, 1965; Eiseman et al, 1963; Horner Andrews et al, 1953; Chung et al, 1962; Kestens and McDermott, 1961; McMenamy et al, 1962; Shoemaker et al, 1960; Kesten et al, 1961). The latter has been used very extensively and has the advantage that much is already known about its physiology. Species differences in response are quite marked in the same viscus. We shall see below for example how the porcine liver behaves in a quite different way to its canine counterpart when some gastro-intestinal hormones are given to it. Clearly differences of this type may on occasions be misleading and perhaps account for the preponderance of interest in the canine and rat livers.

In choosing the animal other factors are important. Much fat particularly in the abdomen of larger animals will increase the surgical difficulties and where this is present the blood vessels seem more easily torn or accidentally injured. For priming a myocardium accustomed to maintaining a high output is desirable. Where dilution of the blood is required for technical reasons there may be an advantage if the animal has a high P.C.V. All of these considerations are met by the greyhound breed. The Weimaranner is also suitable and has the advantage of having fewer blood group incompatibilities. Most of our work is done on the former. Their average weight is 25 kg.

Where pigs are to be used size is important and here also we recommend animals weighing around 25 kg. Pigs have the disadvantage that they are technically more difficult to anaesthetise. For studies on the biliary tree, however, they are to be preferred to the dog. The porcine bile ducts and sphincter are much more like the human.

References

Andrews, W.H.H., Hecker, R. and Maegraith, B.G. (1956) The action of adrenaline, noradrenaline, acetylcholine and histamine on the perfused liver of the monkey, cat and rabbit. *J. Physiol,* **132,** 509.

Brauer, R.W., Pessotti, R.L. and Pizzolato, P. (1951) Isolated rat liver preparation. Bile production and other basic properties. *Proc. Soc. Exp. Biol. Med.* **78,** 174.

Burton, S.D., St. George, S. and Ishida, T. (1960) Small volume perfusion system of the isolated rat liver. *J. Appl. Physiol.* **15,** 128.

Chapman, N.D., Goldsworth, P.D., Volwiler, W., *et al.* (1961) The isolated perfused bovine liver. *J. Exp. Med.* **113,** 981.

Chapman, N.D., Goldsworthy, P.D., Nyhus, L.M., *et al.* (1960) Studies in isolated organ physiology: bromsulphalein clearance in the isolated perfused bovine liver. *Surgery* **48,** 111.

Chung, W.B., Moore, J.R. and Mersereau, W. (1962) A technique of isolated perfusion of the liver. *Surgery* **51,** 508.

Corey, E.L. and Britton, S.W. (1941) Glycogen levels in the isolated liver perfused with cortico-adrenal extract, insulin and other preparations. *Amer. J. Physiol.* **131,** 783.

Craig, A.B. Jr., (1959) Effects of epinephrine on lactic and keto-acid production, phosphate balance and pH changes in the isolated perfused frog liver. *Amer. J. Physiol.* **196,** 969.

Craig, A.B. Jr. (1958) Observations on epinephrine and glucagon-induced glycogenolysis and potassium loss in the isolated perfused frog liver. *Amer. J. Physiol.* **193,** 425.

Craig, A.B. Jr. (1959) Effects of iodoacetate on potassium, glucose and lactic acid metabolism in isolated perfused frog liver. *Amer. J. Physiol.* **197,** 289.

Eiseman, B., Knipe, P., Koh, Y., *et al.* (1963) Factors affecting hepatic vascular resistance in the perfused liver. *Ann. Surg.* **157,** 532.

Eiseman, B., Knipe, P., McColl, H., *et al.* (1961) Isolated liver perfusion for reducing blood ammonia. *Arch Surg.* (Chicago) **83,** 356.

Eiseman, B., Moore, T.C. and Normell, L. (1964) Histamine metabolism on the isolated perfused pig liver. *Surg. Gynec. Obstet.* **118,** 69.

Gunberg, D.L., Lyons, W.R. and Johnson, R.E. (1961) Perfusion studies of the isolated young rat liver. *J. Lab. Clin. Med.* **45,** 130.

Hardcastle, J.D. and Ritchie, H.D. (1967) The liver in shock. *Brit. J. Surg.* **54,** 679.

Hardcastle, J.D. and Ritchie, H.D. (1968) The liver in shock. *Brit. J. Surg.* **55,** 365.

Hardcastle, J.D. (1965) Glucose and potassium levels in the isolated perfused canine liver. M. Chir. Thesis (Cantab.).

Horner Andrews, W.H., Hecker, R., Maegraith, B.G., and Ritchie, H.D. (1953) Technique of perfusion of the canine liver. *J. Physiol.* **122,** 9 Proceedings.

Kestens, P.J., Farrelly, J.A. and McDermott, W.V. (1961) A technique of isolation and perfusion of the canine liver. *J. Surg. Res.* **1,** 58.

Kestens, P.J. and McDermott, W.V. Jr. (1961) Perfusion and replacement of the canine liver. *Surgery* **50,** 196.

Lundsgaard, E. (1938) The metabolism of the isolated liver. *Bull Hopkins Hosp.* **63,** 90.

McCarthy, R.D., Shaw, J.C. and Lakshmanan, S. (1958) Metabolism of volatile fatty acids by the perfused goat liver. *Proc. Soc. Exp. Biol. Med.* **99,** 560.

McMenamy, R.H., Shoemaker, W.C., Richmond, J.E., *et al.* (1962) Uptake and metabolism of amino-acids by the dog liver perfused *in situ. Amer. J. Physiol.* **202,** 407.

Miller, L.L., Bly, C.G., Watson, M.L., *et al.* (1951) The dominant role of the liver in plasma protein synthesis. *J. Exp. Med.* **94,** 431.

Mortimore, G.E. (1961) Effect of insulin on potassium transfer in isolated rat liver. *Amer. J. Physiol.* **200,** 1315.

Price, J.B. Jr. and Dietrich, L.S. (1957) The induction of tryptophan peroxidase in the isolated perfused liver. *J. Biol. Chem.* **227,** 633.

Shoemaker, W.C., Panico, F.G., Walker, W.F., *et al.* (1960) Perfusion of canine liver *in vivo. J. Appl. Physiol.* **15,** 687.

Young, M.K. Jr., Prudden, J.F. and Stirman, J.A. (1955) A perfusion technique for the study of liver metabolism. *J. Lab. Clin. Med.* **46,** 155.

CHAPTER FOUR
Anaesthesia

Isolation and perfusion of an organ of the gastro-intestinal tract involves considerable surgical preparation under general anaesthesia. It is essential that the anaesthetic technique adopted does not have significant adverse effects on gastro-intestinal tract function, either during the surgical procedure or subsequently on the completed preparation. These adverse effects may arise in two main ways: firstly the splanchnic circulation may be reduced by general factors such as hypotension, hypoxia, changes in acid-base and fluid balance, and increased circulating catecholamines; secondly, the splanchnic circulation and the function of the gastro-intestinal tract organs may be depressed as a direct result of the anaesthetic drugs used. These problems however may be reduced by avoidance of overdosage, careful attention to technique and adequate monitoring.

Anaesthesia may be regarded as a triad of unconsciousness, analgesia and muscular relaxation when appropriate. To this end, unconsciousness is most commonly induced by intravenous injection of drugs such as barbiturates, or inhalation of volatile agents. Maintenance and control of level of anaesthesia is best achieved by inhalation of volatile agents. Intermittent, incremental intravenous injections lead to undesirable variations in depth of anaesthesia. Ventilation may be either spontaneous or controlled.

Disposable syringes and needles should be used. These have the advantages of sterility, and the risk of infection to the investigator is reduced.

Ideally a Boyle's (continuous flow) anaesthetic machine should be available. Oxygen and nitrous oxide should be delivered to the animal through a calibrated, temperature-compensated vaporiser for volatile agents, with the flow rate controlled by rotameters. A standard Magill circuit with reservoir bag and Heidbrink valve is suitable for spontaneous ventilation.

Simple, automatic mechanical ventilators suitable for animals are available, such as the Palmer or Harvard systems. However any of the machines in clinical use is acceptable, provided that appropriate tidal volumes and a wide range of ventilatory rate can be achieved. In general terms, relatively large tidal volumes and low respiratory rates have the advantage of preventing areas of collapse in the lung. Care should be taken to avoid rebreathing when intermittent positive pressure ventilation (IPPV) is instituted (Mushin *et al*, 1969). It is also a wise precaution to check apparatus before use for leaks, appropriate connections of tubes, etc. In addition, it should be ascertained that the machine is suitable for anaesthetic gases.

Standard cuffed red rubber or plastic endotracheal tubes are available in a range of sizes suitable for most animals. The cuff should always be checked before use. A problem which may arise is one of length. The tubes should be used uncut, as supplied by the manufacturer, and if necessary an extension fitted for long-necked animals.

Initial Preparation

Animals, like man, withstand anaesthesia and surgery best when fit. For this reason every effort should be made to ensure that the animals used are disease free and well nourished. If possible, to avoid the hazard of vomiting during induction of anaesthesia, animals should not be fed on the night prior to surgery. However, prolonged starvation leads to glycogen depletion of the liver and may interact adversely with anaesthesia (Biebuyck and Alberti, 1972). Premedication is not usually indicated, as most of the suitable drugs depress the cardiovascular system and remain in the tissues for prolonged periods. Atropine however may be given intramuscularly, as a drying agent, if difficulty with intubation is anticipated.

Induction of Anaesthesia

(a)   Intravenous injection

This is the simplest method of inducing anaesthesia in large animals. The dose should be calculated on a weight basis and injected slowly to avoid undue cardiorespiratory depression. Suitable veins, depending on the animal, may be found on the dorsal aspect of the ear, in the limbs, in the neck and in the tail.

Of the drugs in common use the short-acting barbiturate, thio-pentone sodium, is probably most suitable. In solution, however, it is extremely alkaline (pH 11) and therefore irritant if injected extra-vascularly. The recently introduced intravenous steroid agent Althesin may have advantages as it is rapidly metabolised and is non-irritant (Child et al, 1971, Savege et al, 1971). Although animals tolerate large doses of barbiturates, relative overdosage causes cardio-respiratory depression. Longer acting barbiturates may also affect the gastro-intestinal tract directly; for example pentobarbitone sodium has been shown to reduce gastric secretion (Merendino, 1948; Sky-ring et al, 1961) and to inhibit motor activity of the bowel (Walker et al, 1956; Gruber et al, 1941; and Quigley et al, 1934). Since barbiturate metabolism by the liver is a slow process some of the drug will almost certainly be incorporated into the perfusion circuit. For this reason, in addition to effects on the donor, the dose of barbiturate should be kept to a minimum.

(b)   Intraperitoneal injection

For convenience this route is employed in small animals where intravenous injection is impractical. The dose should be calculated on a weight basis and care taken to avoid damage to the gastro-intestinal tract during injection. It should be remembered that the intraperi-toneal route may lead to very high concentrations of drugs being presented to the liver. Under these circumstances, damage may be produced in the liver which is not seen with dosing by more orthodox routes.

Medium acting barbiturates such as pentobarbitone sodium are most frequently used for intraperitoneal injection, as no further anaesthesia is then required. Care should be taken to avoid respira-tory obstruction after induction and during surgery.

(c)   Intramuscular injection

This route is suitable for larger animals where handling is difficult. A long sharp needle should be used to ensure correct injection and facilities should be available for restraint during the induction period.

Barbiturates are not ideally suited for intramuscular injection as correct dosage may be difficult to calculate and induction time is variable. Recently Roberts (1971) has described the use of intramuscular ketamine hydrochloride in pigs, using a pistol and dart. Ketamine, in addition to its anaesthetic properties, is a cardiovascular stimulant leading to a rise in both pulse rate and blood pressure. The exact mechanism of these cardiovascular effects is unknown as is its effect on the splanchnic circulation.

(d)   Inhalation – Volatile agents

Induction by inhalation is in general less satisfactory than by injection. There is the difficulty of obtaining an air-tight fit with a mask, although special 'snout' masks are available. In addition, struggling during induction will lead to catecholamine release and even injury to the animal or inexperienced personnel.

Of the volatile agents available halothane is most suitable. It should always be administered using a calibrated vaporiser designed specifically for halothane. Other vaporisers or simple bottles may lead to overdosage which is associated with marked cardiovascular depression in most animal species. 3–4% halothane may be needed for induction, but the concentration should be reduced as soon as possible once the animal is asleep and 0·5–1% is usually adequate for maintenance, especially if nitrous oxide is used in addition. The motility of the jejunum, colon and stomach in dogs is depressed by halothane, but activity returns promptly after the agent is discontinued (Marshall, 1961).

Halothane affects the cardiovascular system by producing peripheral vasodilation and myocardial depression. Catecholamine secretion is suppressed. Thus, provided cardiac output does not fall, the splanchnic circulation will be maintained. In contrast, diethyl ether and cyclopropane stimulate the release of catecholamines, leading to a reduction in the splanchnic circulation. In addition, both these agents are inflammable in air and explosive when mixed with oxygen: an important consideration in animal laboratories which may not be spark-proof. For these reasons, diethyl ether and cyclopropane are not suitable during surgery for gastro-intestinal tract perfusion studies.

Maintenance of Anaesthesia

After induction, anaesthesia should be maintained at a light level, compatible with the surgery, thus avoiding cardiovascular depression.

B

However, inadequate anaesthesia is associated with catecholamine release, which may be compounded by concomitant hypoxia and a raised arterial PCO_2 ($PaCO_2$) due to inadequate ventilation. This combination reduces splanchnic blood flow with detrimental effect on the gastro-intestinal tract.

To control these problems the airway must be secured, if possible by intubation or tracheostomy. If spontaneous ventilation is inadequate, as judged by a rising arterial PCO_2, or the chest is opened, intermittent positive pressure ventilation should be instituted to maintain the $PaCO_2$ at approximately 40 mm Hg.

Nitrous oxide (N_2O) has a minimal effect on the cardiovascular system and is a good analgesic. It has the advantage of rapid excretion and because it is poorly soluble it helps, as does nitrogen, to maintain stability of the lung. It is, however, a weak anaesthetic even at high concentration. In practice, the risk of hypoxia limits the use of nitrous oxide to a 70:30 mixture with oxygen. Such a mixture should produce an adequate arterial PO_2 (PaO_2, 100–200 mm Hg). Higher oxygen levels (arterial PO_2 > 300 mm Hg) should be avoided as arterial vasoconstriction occurs, which may affect gastro-intestinal tract function.

In summary, anaesthesia may be maintained in most large animals by either spontaneous or intermittent positive pressure ventilation, via an endotracheal tube, with nitrous oxide and oxygen. If necessary, a low concentration of halothane may be added to the mixture or additional intravenous agent given.

Muscle relaxants

Adequate muscular relaxation and control of ventilation can usually be achieved in animals without the use of muscle relaxants. Furthermore, in accordance with the Cruelty to Animals Act (1876), written permission is required from the Secretary of State before any muscle relaxant may be administered to an animal even in combination with other anaesthetic drugs. In addition, forty-eight hours' notice of each individual experiment must be given to the Home Office, to enable an inspector to be present if this is considered necessary by the Secretary of State.

Suxamethonium, a short-acting depolarising agent, has been used to facilitate intubation in pigs (Fowler *et al*, 1962); under these circumstances, however, hypoxia is inevitable unless intubation is performed rapidly. The long-acting curare-like non-depolarising muscle relaxants, other than pancuronium bromide, lead to histamine release and ganglion blockade which may cause arterial hypotension (see Chapter 8 for effects on the canine liver). Also, many of these drugs are protein bound and may therefore be incorporated into the perfusion circuit.

Monitoring during anaesthesia

Where possible, arterial and central venous pressure, temperature and acid-base balance should be monitored during surgery. Arterial pressure is best measured by a cannula in a peripheral artery connected to either a mercury- or electromanometer. The cannula may also be used for withdrawing arterial blood samples for gas analysis of PO_2, PCO_2, pH and bicarbonate in addition to any other base-line measurements which may be relevant to the subsequent perfusion study.

Central venous pressure (CVP) may be measured by a cannula placed in the right atrium, inserted via a peripheral vein and then connected to either a saline or electromanometer. The zero of the manometer is adjusted level with the assumed height of the heart and there should be a clear rise and fall in central venous pressure in time with ventilation. A fall in central venous pressure may be associated with loss of circulating blood volume and should be treated by infusion. The choice of fluid depends on the circumstances. Blood is ideal but may not be available, perfusate diluent is the next choice and failing this dextran plasma expanding solutions or dextrose or dextrose-saline solutions should be used. Transient changes in arterial pressure and central venous pressure may be associated with surgical manoeuvres and care should be taken to reduce such incidents to a minimum.

Body temperature of the animal should be measured and the laboratory itself maintained at a reasonable ambient temperature, since heat loss is particularly associated with gastro-intestinal surgery. If body temperature falls, temperature correction factors will need to be applied for blood gas measurements (Kelman and Nunn, 1966). In addition, a marked fall in body temperature will lead to cardiovascular depression and possibly to cardiac arrest. A warming blanket or external heating may therefore be required. Similarly, if massive transfusion is anticipated arrangements should be made for warming the infusion fluid. Animal temperature is best measured by either an oesophageal or rectal probe connected to a remote temperature gauge. Glass thermometers should be avoided to prevent injury to either the animal or the investigator.

Acid-base changes often occur during surgical procedures in

animals. The respiratory component is readily controlled by intermittent positive pressure ventilation and oxygen administration. Ideally, arterial PCO_2 should be maintained at approximately 40 mm Hg. Metabolic acidosis, manifest as a low arterial pH and standard bicarbonate, may be associated with hypotension or excessive handling of the gastro-intestinal tract. Severe metabolic acidosis (pH less than 7·2) will produce cardiovascular depression. Such an acidosis should be corrected by the infusion of sodium bicarbonate ($NaHCO_3$) solution. 1·4% $NaHCO_3$ solution is isotonic and contains 1 mEq in 6 ml. Stronger solutions are available, up to 8·4% $NaHCO_3$, i.e. 1 mEq per ml, but these are of course hypertonic and may be inappropriate.

Since most surgical preparations involve some fluid loss it is advantageous, where practical, to routinely provide fluid replacement. Additional therapy should be guided by the arterial and central venous pressures, and acid-base status.

Techniques in Common Laboratory Animals

(a)   The rat

Anaesthesia is most easily induced by intraperitoneal injection, e.g. pentobarbitone sodium (80 mg/kg). In skilled hands the tail vein may be used for intravenous injection. One dose of barbiturate is usually adequate as surgical preparation time is short. The airway may be controlled by tongue traction.

(b)   The dog

Intravenous induction is readily performed using a front leg vein. Prior to injection, the skin should be shaved if necessary and a muzzle is a wise precaution if the handler is inexperienced. Thiopentone sodium 15–25 mg/kg is a reasonable induction dose.

Intubation may be performed under barbiturate anaesthesia – muscle relaxants are not required. The dog should be placed on its side on the operating table, the mouth is then opened and the tongue pulled out over the lower jaw with a gauze swab. An assistant elevates the upper jaw. The epiglottis should now be visible and an endotracheal tube may be passed over it into the larynx. In 25–30 kg dogs 9–10 mm internal diameter, uncut cuffed Magill endotracheal tubes are suitable. Once in position, the cuff should be inflated and the tube carefully secured.

(c)   The pig

In animals weighing less than 50 kg, the dorsal aspect of the ear is a suitable site for intravenous injection. Alternatively, anaesthesia may be induced with halothane using a snout mask. In the larger pig, intravenous or intramuscular injection is more suitable. Barbiturates, (Vaughan, 1961, Berman *et al*, 1970), ketamine (Roberts, 1971) or phencylclidine (Taverner, 1963) may be used. Intramuscular atropine 1 mg reduces salivation and may facilitate intubation.

The airway is difficult to maintain in an unconscious pig. The tongue should be pulled well forward and the head extended as far as possible. Intubation is not a simple procedure and suxamethonium 1 mg/kg intravenously may be advantageous (Fowler *et al*, 1962; Roberts, 1971). The pig is placed on its back or side and an assistant holds down the upper jaw, snout and upper lips. The tongue is pulled out with a gauze swab and traction applied to elevate the lower jaw. A long laryngoscope (Roberts, 1971) is inserted and used either to elevate or displace the epiglottis until the entrance of the larynx is visualised. A variety of sizes of cuffed endotracheal tubes and a wire introducer should be available as it is difficult to assess the tracheal size from the pig itself. As a rough guide, in pigs weighing 30–50 kg it is difficult to insert an endotracheal tube with an internal diameter of greater than 6–7 mm. The intubating position described in the pig is somewhat different from that encountered in man. It may be helpful for those familiar only with the latter, if in the pig they reverse the normal direction in inserting an endotracheal tube such that the curvature initially faces backwards rather than forwards. Once past the vocal cords the tube is rotated to its usual position.

Certain strains of pigs may develop malignant hyperthermia under anaesthesia (Berman *et al*, 1970). This is manifest as a rapidly increasing body temperature, usually muscular rigidity, severe metabolic acidosis and hyperkalaemia. The condition is most commonly associated with halothane and the muscle relaxant suxamethonium, although it has been reported with other anaesthetic agents. Once the condition is fully developed it is invariably fatal. Withdrawal of the anaesthetic, energetic cooling, alkali therapy and procaine amide in large doses may reverse the condition in its early stages (Harrison, 1971). As malignant hyperthermia is an hereditary condition litter mates are often affected.

References

Berman, M.C., Harrison, G.G., Bull, A.B. and Kench, J.E. (1970) Changes underlying halothane induced malignant hyperpyrexia in Landrace pigs. *Nature* **225**, 653.

Biebuyck, J.F. and Alberti, K.G.M.M. (1972) The effect of anaesthetic agents on carbohydrate metabolism in the rat. *Clin. Sci.* **42**, 4.

Child, K.J., Currie, J.P., Davis, B., Dodds, M.G., Pearce, D.R. and Twissell, D.J. (1971) The pharmacological properties in animals of CT1341 – a new steroid anaesthetic agent. *Brit. J. Anaes.* **43**, 2.

Fowler, J., Hill, D.W., Morgan, R.L., Nunn, J.F., Weaver, B. and Woolmer, R.F. (1962) Anaesthesia for the irradiated pig: A study in remote control. *Anaesthesia* **34**, 327.

Gruber, C.M. and Gruber, C.M. Jr. (1941) The effect of barbituric and thiobarbituric acid derivatives on the pyloric sphincter and stomach in unanaesthetised dogs. *J. Pharmacol. Exp. Ther.* **72**, 176.

Harrison, G.G. (1971) Anaesthetic-induced malignant hyperpyrexia: A suggested method of treatment. *Brit. Med. J.* **3**, 454.

Kelman, G.R. and Nunn, J.F. (1966) Nomograms for correction of blood PO_2, PCO_2, pH and base excess for time and temperature. *J. Appl. Physiol.* **21**, 1484.

Marshall, F.N. (1961) Effects of halothane on gastrointestinal motility. *Anaesthesiology* **22**, 363.

Merendino, K.A. (1948) The effect of pentobarbital on the gastric secretion in dog and man. *Gastroenterology* **10**, 531.

Mushin, W.W., Rendell-Baker, L., Thompson, P.W. and Mapleson, W.W. (1969) *Automatic ventilation of the lungs*. Second Edn. Blackwell Scientific Publications, Oxford and Edinburgh.

Quigley, J.P. and Phelps, K.R. (1934) Observations regarding the mechanism of gastrointestinal inhibition by barbituric acid compounds. *J. Pharmacol. Exp. Ther.* **50**, 420.

Roberts, F.W. (1971) Anaesthesia for pigs (Intramuscular ketamine as an induction agent). *Anaesthesia* **26**, 445.

Savege, T.M., Foley, E.I., Coultas, R.J., Walton, B., Strunin, L., Simpson, B.R. and Scott, D.F. (1971) CT1341: some effects in man. Cardiorespiratory, electro-encephalographic and biochemical measurements. *Anaesthesia* **26**, 4.

Skyring, A.P., Milton, G.W. and Maxwell, G.A. (1961) Effect of sodium pentobarbital on histamine stimulated gastric secretion. *Amer. J. Physiol.* **201**, 574.

Taverner, W.D. (1963) A study of the effect of phencyclidine in the pig. *Vet. Rec.* **75,** 1377.

Vaughan, L.C. (1961) Anaesthesia in the pig. *Br. Vet. J.* **117,** 383.

Walker, L. and Necheles, H. (1956) Inhibition by barbiturates of barium-stimulated intestinal motility. *Amer. J. Physiol.* **185,** 624.

CHAPTER FIVE

Apparatus

The purpose of this section is to describe and discuss the merits of the great variety of standard equipment available, including that which may be easily manufactured by a department workshop, for perfusion experiments. It will cover the basic standing apparatus: trolleys, water baths, organ chambers and so on; the choice of pumps, oxygenators, and heat exchangers; and finally the use of tubing, connectors and other ancillary fittings to the perfusion circuit itself.

Standing Equipment

The basic essential for perfusion work is a mobile trolley on which all the apparatus for the experiment may be mounted. For small animal work such as the rat liver perfusion, it should ideally incorporate the operating area close to the perfusion circuit; for experiments with the dog or pig, the requirements should be tailored to the position and height of the operating table on which the surgical procedure will be performed.

The trolley should house the perfusion circuit itself, reservoir, oxygenator and pump, water bath and organ chamber and a certain amount of extra space for the placement of small additional items of equipment. The entire structure should be as simple as possible, free from sharp corners, and easily cleaned. There should be no access for blood and secretions to undersurfaces, cavities or recesses where they may be missed during cleaning. Height is important and has bearing upon the animal under study and the type of experiment to be performed. There must always be free venous drainage from the operating table to the perfusion trolley, and from the organ chamber to the reservoir or oxygenator. Below the working top there may be incorporated gas cylinders to supply the oxygenator, and further space to accommodate additional items of monitoring equipment. This latter aspect of the design is one of individual preference and requirement and needs no further discussion. Finally, it is useful to incorporate into the basic design of the trolley itself an electrically safe power supply, able to accommodate all the perfusion and monitoring equipment. This avoids the inconvenient and often hazardous procedure of leading multiple power cables away to wall plugs.

Organ Chamber

The perfused preparation must be maintained at a constant temperature and humidity, usually 38°C. However, conditions may be varied to suit the protocol of the experiment. A chamber is required, to provide a stable external environment, and the blood must be warm before it enters to maintain the core temperature of the organ. A large water bath incorporating a thermostat unit provides an ideal heat source, and is preferred to the use of infra-red lamps which are more difficult to control, and exert a considerable drying effect on the preparation.

There are available disposable plastic chambers for use in perfusion experiments, which may be suspended in a water bath; these provide ideal environmental control but are less satisfactory if access to the preparation is required for visualisation or recording purposes.

A small perspex box with a lid provides a simple solution to the problem, but the surface on which the preparation rests is hard, and may cause tissue damage by prolonged pressure on one site. Temperature control is not so precise. A third alternative we prefer is to incorporate a chamber into the top of the water bath itself. Figure 3 shows the design of such a chamber. Over part of a relatively large (20 litre) water bath is stretched a thin sheet of polythene upon which the organ rests, its weight supported by the fluid underneath. A second sheet of polythene sealed with saline at the edges covers the preparation, and a perspex cover completes the insulation, while at the same time permitting visualisation and direct access if required.

This design has proved satisfactory for most of the preparations described in later chapters. Blood flow to a small organ such as the stomach or pancreas, however, is not sufficient to maintain a constant temperature in the face of external heat loss, and a special chamber for these preparations is essential. In the liver, temperature control depends largely on the blood flow to the viscus, and is ensured by effective heating of the perfusing blood itself.

Heat Exchangers

It is not usual to maintain the oxygenator and reservoir at 38°C in perfusion work, although this has been done in the case of the pancreas and gallbladder (Chapter 10).

A heat exchanger is therefore required in the arterial side of the circuit. This should have as small a priming volume as is compatible with adequate heat transfer, and its size and configuration will depend upon the flow rate, and the temperature of the blood. For all small organ perfusions in which the blood flow rate is less than 200 cc/min, and the temperature differential less than 10°C, some form of disposable PVC coil immersed in the water bath is satisfactory. For higher flow rates, as in liver perfusion work, a stainless steel water jacket type of heat exchanger may be necessary. A high circulating flow rate in the water jacket will ensure adequate heating of the blood. All heat exchangers by virtue of their relatively large internal volume provide a trap for bubbles. It is important that these are all removed, prior to the initiation of perfusion, or air embolisation will occur.

Pumps

All pumps damage circulating blood. The amount of damage depends on the type of pump, on the flow rate, and the number of pumping strokes per minute. The maximum use should be made of gravity in allowing blood to be transferred passively from one part of the perfusion system to another, and ideally pumps should only be used for the final arterial input. The pump should be calibrated in such a way that, at any given setting, output is constant over the physiological range of perfusion pressures, 60 – 160 mm Hg. Thus since the output is known, changes in the vascular resistance of the organ can be inferred by any change in perfusion pressure, since the flow rate has remained the same.

For actual perfusion, pumping is better than a gravity system in which the pressure head remains constant and flow may vary continuously with changes in the vascular resistance, which may only be detected by continuous monitoring with an accurate flow meter.

Flow and not pressure is of prime importance in this type of work, a consideration which makes the use of calibrated pumps essential as being the simplest and most reliable way of controlling this aspect of the perfusion. The addition of an electromagnetic flow meter permits direct recording of flow and allows precise studies to be undertaken. In isolated organs satisfactory arterial perfusion, as judged by other criteria (see Monitoring) is usually achieved at a pressure of between 60 and 80 mm Hg. Liver preparations, however, require the addition of portal venous perfusion, and this is maintained at pressure of 8 – 10 cm H_2O. This low pressure range, as compared with the intact

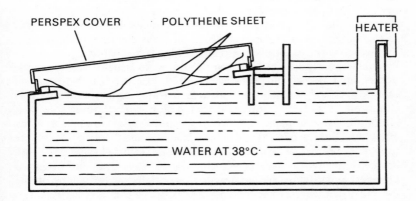

PERSPEX COVER   POLYTHENE SHEET   HEATER

WATER AT 38°C

Fig. 3 Water bath/organ chamber. Using a large water bath as a source of heat the perfused organ may be maintained at a constant temperature and humidity by enclosing it between two layers of thin polythene sheet. The water provides a soft bed upon which the organ rests, and ripples at the interface prevent pressure necrosis and venous obstruction.

animal, may be due to denervation, dilution of the perfusate and the lack of circulating catecholamines which are rapidly taken up by the preparations and inactivated.

Choice of pump is based firstly on size and it should have, over its optimal working range, an output of 0 – 150 ml/min for stomach and other small viscus perfusions, and 0 – 400 ml/min for liver perfusions; secondly, it depends on the characteristics of the flow induced by the pump. For perfusion of the portal vein in the liver, for instance, non-pulsatile flow is required. This may, of course, be achieved by a gravity feed system, with the disadvantages already described, or a simple screw non-pulsatile pump may be used. As an alternative, the flow from any pulsatile pump may be 'depulsed' by the addition of a closed side-arm to the arterial line in which is trapped a column of air. The length of the column required to damp the pulse width to zero for any given values of flow and pressure is easily determined by experiment.

Some consideration must also be given to the question of pulsatile or non-pulsatile flow in the arterial perfusion. Brodie in 1903 discussing the perfusion of surviving organs argued that perfusions should be pulsatile for teleological reasons, and noted that the development of oedema in a perfused organ was minimised by pulsatile flow. Later Hooker (1910) attempted to relate kidney function to the type of perfusion and performed experiments using various flow characteristics all at a constant mean pressure. He observed that the amount of filtrate produced by the kidney was related directly to the pulse pressure, whereas the volume of protein lost was subject to an inverse relationship. Here then was one organ which, when studied in isolation, appeared to benefit from pulsatile perfusion. Parsons and McMaster (1938) studied lymph formation and flow in the rabbit's ear and demonstrated clearly that this was enhanced by pulsatile flow, and that if flow was non-pulsatile then lymph flow was impaired and local oedema would accumulate. They attributed this in part to the purely mechanical deformation of the walls of small vessels by the pulse. Giron et al (1966) used a depulsing device implanted in parallel with the aorta of the dog, and observed changes in systemic blood pressure associated with failure of the carotid baroreceptor mechanism to respond to a non-pulsatile mean pressure.

More recently there have been a number of studies in both the experimental animal and man of the beneficial effects of pulsatile flow in relation to whole-body perfusion. Comparisons were between the damped sine-wave pulse produced by a roller pump and a pulse trace designed to resemble that in the aorta. During periods of 2 hours cardio-pulmonary by-pass in dogs Trinkel et al (1968) observed decreased vascular resistance, higher flow rates and diminished lactate production during pulsatile perfusion. Shepherd and Kirklin (1969) also found decreased peripheral vascular resistance and significantly improved tissue oxygen consumption during four hours cardio-pulmonary by-pass in calves when using a pulsatile pump. Jacobs et al (1969) studied renal function, peripheral vascular resistance and lactate production in dogs subjected to extended periods of left heart by-pass using a pulsatile pump. They observed a significant increase in urine volume and creatinine clearance, less of a tendency for the peripheral vascular resistance to rise, and a marked reduction in lactic acidaemia. Pulsatile cardio-pulmonary by-pass in man has been

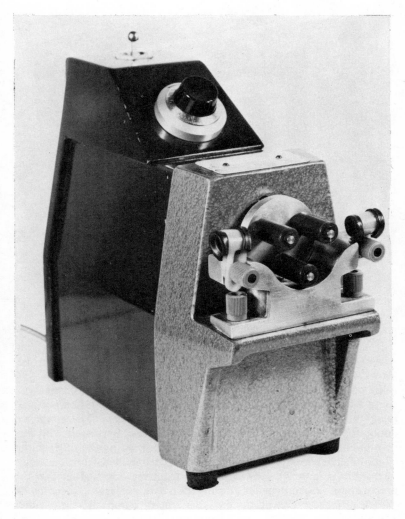

Fig. 4 The Watson Marlow pump. A small roller pump suitable for organ perfusion work.

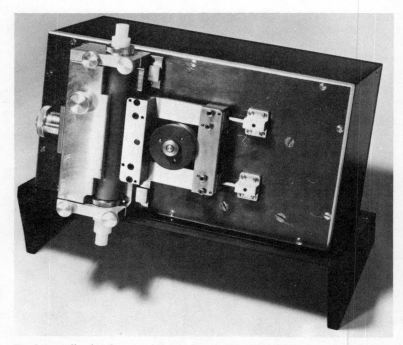

Fig. 5 A small pulsatile pump designed for organ perfusion. The output may be varied by increasing the stroke volume or the rate.

shown by Trinkel *et al* (1971) to be associated with similar improvements.

In our laboratory isolated organ perfusion has been carried out using a roller pump (Figure 4) obtained commercially, and a pulsatile pump built in the department workshop (Figure 5). There was no doubt that the pressure tracing obtained during perfusion with our own pump was an improvement on that produced by the roller pump (Figure 6). It closely approximated to that obtained from the dog's own aorta (Figure 7). However, apart from the observation that the preparations looked 'better' during pulsatile perfusion, there is no evidence at the present time, that this type of pump offers any other advantage over the occlusive roller pump. That it is so may be related to the denervation of these isolated preparations with, therefore, no tendency for a progressive neurogenic shut-down of the peripheral circulation to occur. Certainly no rise in perfusion pressure was observed with either type of pump, even after 4 or 5 hours.

ROLLER PUMP

seconds
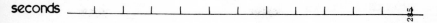

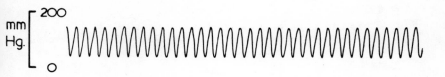

PULSATILE PUMP

seconds
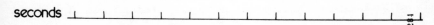

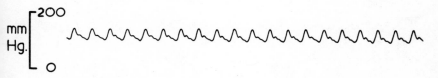

Fig. 6 The characteristics of the pulse in the perfusion cannula obtained with a roller pump (top trace), and pulsatile pump (bottom trace). Both were perfusing the same circuit and organ at comparable flow rates.

Is it therefore necessary to use pulsatile pumps in the present context? They have of course several disadvantages, being usually complex, expensive and traumatic to blood. In addition they are not at present readily available. By contrast, the more usual type of roller pump is simple, reliable and relatively inexpensive. It does not, however, reproduce a physiological period of systolic and diastolic pressure, but a sinusoidal pulse distributed about a mean. There are a great variety available and one with the appropriate output for an experimental programme is readily obtained.

GREYHOUND AORTA

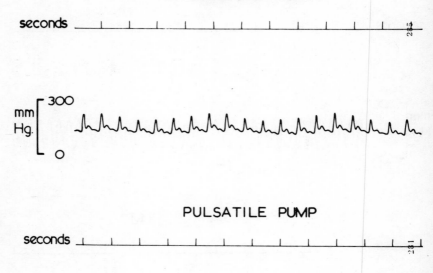

PULSATILE PUMP

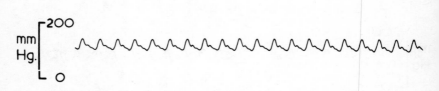

Fig. 7 Pulsatile flow in the dog and the perfusion system.

In summary, we would advocate for routine use an occlusive roller pump for its simplicity and effectiveness. It must be of a size appropriate to the flow required: it is of no value to have a small pump turning at 200 rpm in an effort to provide adequate flow. The pulse rate is unphysiological and the blood damage considerable. Too large a pump, on the other hand, may have to be run so slowly that output becomes inaccurate. It must be possible to adjust the occlusion of the rollers accurately to minimise blood damage. However, the use of a pulsatile pump is recommended when studies on the vascular system are planned. The responses to vaso-active drugs, which are always brisk in isolated preparations, may well be influenced by the character of the pulse pressure, as may be the actual distribution of blood flow to the various tissue compartments.

Regardless of the type of pump used the pulse pressure should also be considered. Blood pumped down a system of PVC tubing and connectors into a small artery undergoes fairly violent changes in pressure and velocity. There is a little compliance in the walls of the circuit under these conditions and the physical changes are transmitted, almost unattenuated, into the arterioles of the organ. This may lead to trauma evidenced as petechial haemorrhages under the serosa, even frank haematoma formation in the omentum of the stomach, blood-stained secretion from mucosal haemorrhage, mucosal oedema, ascites from the liver surface and blood-stained bile. To offset these changes a compliance should be introduced into the circuit. A side-arm filled with a column of air is adequate and the volume of air required is easily determined by experiment. The top of the column may be conveniently connected to an aneroid pressure gauge for monitoring perfusion pressure. This method is useful when smaller arteries are cannulated directly as for example during pancreatic perfusion (Chapter 10). An alternative, which is preferable for intestinal perfusions, is to cannulate the aorta, incorporating approximately 5 centimetres of it into the circuit. This provides a good elastic compliance and is important in the development of truly pulsatile perfusion, since the contribution of any pump to flow ceases with the closure of its valve at the end of a 'systole'. A mean perfusion pressure of 60–80 mm Hg with a pulse pressure of up to 40 mm Hg will be found to provide adequate flow for most intestinal preparations with minimal evidence of trauma to the vascular structure.

Oxygenators

Accurate control of perfusate gas tensions is an essential feature of all isolated organ studies and is achieved by the incorporation of an oxygenator into the perfusion circuit. All oxygenators cause some damage to the blood which passes through them, either by the action of a direct blood gas interface, or by the exposure of the blood to a large surface area of synthetic membrane.

The choice first of all, therefore, must be for an oxygenator of sufficient size, and no more, to cope adequately with the maximum expected flow rate. In this way unnecessary exposure of the blood to trauma is avoided. Furthermore, simplicity and ease of dismantling for cleaning are important. If disposable units are used then cost becomes an important factor. With these considerations in mind the three types of oxygenator currently available will be discussed.

Bubble Oxygenator

In this type of oxygenator a gas mixture is bubbled through the blood and then the oxygenated blood is debubbled and filtered.

Many oxygenators of this type are available, and the small ones are particularly suited to organ perfusion work with low flow rates. The small priming volume is a particular advantage. The oxygenators are made of disposable plastic and, because of large scale manufacturing for use in cardiac surgery, the cost is reasonable. The bubble oxygenator may be conveniently incorporated into a water bath if this is desired.

The major disadvantage of the bubble oxygenator is the blood damage which occurs at high flow rates, particularly in a closed system.

Disc Oxygenator

The method of filming blood on a large surface area and exposing this directly to a gas mixture has been known for a long time. Bjork (1948) described 40 or 50 discs dipping into a trough of blood, the blood being filmed on the discs and renewed after each exposure by continuous rotation. A variation on this principle was described by Miller, Gibbon and Gibbon (1951) in which blood was allowed to flow, under the influence of gravity, down a number of wire gauze screens. The practical difficulty with the latter system was that sometimes streaming of the blood caused the formation of rivulets which resulted in a considerable loss of surface area available for gas exchange.

Of the two methods, the rotating disc oxygenator has proved the most satisfactory, and is ideal in many respects for organ perfusion work. Firstly, it is available commercially in several sizes, and at reasonable cost. Stainless steel and polycarbonate have both been used for construction, and these are both long lasting, easily cleaned and non-toxic materials. Gas exchange is rapid and easily controlled either by changing the gas mixture, or by increasing or decreasing the rotation of the discs. A 6-inch oxygenator, incorporating 40 discs, is adequate for a flow rate of 100 ml/min at 30 rpm, and for 500 ml/min at 100 rpm. The disc oxygenator causes less blood damage than the bubble type but has the disadvantage of requiring a larger priming volume. To reduce damage, the number of plates and their speed of rotation should be the minimum required for adequate oxygenation. The blood level in the oxygenator should be such that the plates enter the blood with the least turbulence and the oxygenator itself should slope gently from venous to arterial end to prevent build-up of blood on the discs. The lower half of the oxygenator may be allowed to stand in a water bath for heating purposes (see Figures 65 and 66).

Roller Oxygenators

The best known of these is perhaps that developed for the Aga Heart-lung machine. This is made up of a tray containing up to six rollers. Blood enters the top or middle of the tray at one of two inlet channels and flows gently downwards being filmed by the rollers as it meets them. The tray is set in an enclosed chamber with a perspex lid. From the lower end it flows into the reservoir which is attached beneath. The rollers are made of perforated plastic and are disposable. The rest of the assembly can be sterilised in ethylene oxide. Single or double concentric rollers can be used and one to six rollers set in the tray. For large subjects more than one tray can be used.

We have found this to be a very atraumatic oxygenator and recommend it particularly for liver perfusion experiments. As usual it is gassed with 95% O_2 and 5% PO_2 but anaesthetic and other gases can be admitted to the chamber.

More details are given in a subsequent chapter (Liver Perfusion).

Membrane Oxygenators

Theoretically the ideal oxygenator is one in which a membrane separates blood from gas as in the normal lung. The membrane must allow diffusion of oxygen and carbon dioxide in both directions at a rate of about 20 ml per square metre per minute, but be impermeable to blood or gas emboli (Melrose et al, 1958).

With this type of oxygenator blood damage by direct exposure to gas and moving parts is not a problem. However, the effects of a synthetic membrane on the cellular and chemical constituents of blood are as yet incompletely understood.

A number of small membrane oxygenators are available that have been designed for organ perfusion work. They have a small priming volume and a low internal resistance to flow. There is already some evidence that red cell and plasma protein damage is reduced using this type of oxygenator (Lee et al, 1961), an advantage which is applicable not only to physiological studies, but more particularly to long-term preservation of organs. A one square metre unit provides adequate oxygenation for flow rates of up to 500 ml/min. The main disadvantage is the price of each disposable unit, this being 10–15 times the running cost of a re-usable disc oxygenator.

It is important that the oxygenator size should be appropriate for the organ being perfused. If it is too small, gas exchange will be inadequate and hypoxia and hypercapnia will result; if it is too large excessive blood damage will be caused. These criteria apply particularly to the perfusion of very small organs such as the rat liver, and specially small oxygenators may need to be constructed.

Gas Mixtures

Normally oxygen 95% and carbon dioxide 5% should be delivered to the oxygenator with a flow rate sufficient to maintain constant flushing. Care should be taken with membrane oxygenators that excess pressure does not build up on the gas side of the membrane as this may lead to gas emboli on the fluid side. If an adequate $PaCO_2$ cannot be maintained with 5% CO_2, extra carbon dioxide should be added. PCO_2 measurements should allow for temperature differences between the perfusate and the PCO_2 electrode and correction tables should be used if necessary (Kelman and Nunn, 1966). Alterations in carbon dioxide should only be used to adjust the arterial PCO_2 and not to alter the pH. The latter may be controlled by the addition of bicarbonate solution.

The use of 95% oxygen will give high PaO_2 readings, depending on the oxygenator, in the region of 400–500 mm Hg. We have no evidence from our own experience that this is in any way harmful to the perfused organ, but if for any reason lower arterial oxygen tensions are required, the oxygenator may be gassed with air and 5% carbon dioxide.

Anti-foam

Foaming is likely to occur in any oxygenator where moving parts are involved in filming blood, particularly if the movements becomes irregular or excessive, and if bubbles of air become trapped in the blood itself. This problem manifests itself primarily in the disc oxygenator, and the routine use of an anti-foam preparation is advisable if the disc rotation exceeds 50 rpm. Anti-foam A* is used routinely for clinical perfusion and has proved satisfactory for organ perfusion studies. It is sufficient to wipe the discs and the casing of the oxygenator with a thin film of this silicone preparation dissolved in petroleum spirit B.P., and then to remove any excess by thorough

* Silicone MS Anti-foam A, Hopkins and Williams Ltd, Chadwell Heath, Essex.

washing of the circuit with saline prior to priming with blood. Jablonski *et al* (1971) have reported an adverse effect of this substance on the pig liver and prefer a less soluble preparation, M.S. 1100*. However, this has to be baked on to the surface prior to use, and is therefore unsuitable for use with materials other than glass or stainless steel.

Tubing and Circuit Fittings

Damage to the blood is incurred not only during oxygenation and pumping, but also by its passage along the perfusion circuit. For this reason, the tubing, connectors and taps should be carefully selected to reduce to a minimum this adverse effect. Ideally, disposable tubing and fittings should be used which completely removes any risk of contamination with foreign protein. However, suitable taps for pressure monitoring and sampling of blood may not be readily or cheaply available as throw-away units, in which case it may be found more convenient to use stainless steel fittings. These should be thoroughly cleaned between experiments according to the régime given at the end of this chapter.

Tubing

The lengths used to make up the circuit should be as short as possible, and the diameter of the tubing selected on the basis of the pressure and flow within the system. On the low pressure venous side of the preparation, a larger diameter is required if free flow of blood, under the influence of gravity, is not to be obstructed by too great a resistance offered by the tubing. On the arterial side the resistance to flow may be overcome by the action of the pump but it is still important not to use too small a diameter tubing, otherwise turbulence will result in greatly increased resistance and damage to the blood. All these problems may be overcome by the use of tubing of more than adequate bore, but this then has the disadvantage of a disproportionate increase in the priming volume of the circuit.

A guide to the internal diameter of tubing based on the flow rate is shown in Table I.

The choice of material for the tubing lies between silicone rubber and polyvinyl chloride (PVC). Silicone rubber has the advantage of

* Silicone MS Anti-foam A, Hopkins and Williams Ltd, Chadwell Heath, Essex.

being extremely inert, and also by virtue of its elasticity adds some compliance to the arterial side of the circuit. It is however expensive and has a further disadvantage in that it is extremely permeable to gases. If the primed circuit is left at a standstill for more than 15 minutes, small bubbles will be seen to have formed inside the tubing, which must then of course be removed before perfusion can be initiated.

Table 1   The Effect of Tubing Size on
Perfusion Pressure

Distal Arterial Pressure 80 mm Hg		
Flow cc/min	Internal diameter of tubing mm	Pressure drop along 1 meter of tubing mm Hg
75	4	40
100	4	60
150	4	100
200	4	160
150	6	5
300	6	15
400	6	20
300	9	0
400	9	5

PVC tubing is readily available in all of the suggested diameters, and is considerably cheaper. It is to be preferred for routine perfusion work, provided heed is taken of the following points. There have been a number of reports of tissue reactions to polymers, and the attention of the reader is drawn to the review of Little and Parkhouse (1962). Pure PVC is rigid and various additives to soften and stabilise it may be toxic if they lake out of the polymer into the surrounding tissue or blood (Guess and Stetson, 1968). Attention was drawn to the importance of blood as a causative factor in this process by Duke and Vane (1968). They found that PVC exposed to a saline solution did not exhibit the same toxic characteristics and concluded that the protein element of whole blood in some way caused these additives to be laked out of the tubing.

It is important therefore to use PVC tubing that conforms to the highest medical grading, and which has been manufactured without the use of organo-tin stabilisers, and other toxic additives known to be insecurely bound to the polymer. Tissue implantation tests are also likely to have been performed on medical grade tubing, but it may be important to check these facts with the manufacturers. If there is any doubt about the quality of the tubing in use, it is possible to perform a simple test with any perfused intestinal viscus as the test object.

PVC Toxicity Test

A metre of the tubing under test is cut into short lengths, and exposed to a 200 ml aliquot of blood from the perfusion circuit for two hours. This should be done under sterile conditions at 37°C, with control samples of blood available for comparison. After the incubation period, 10 ml samples are injected into the arterial side of the perfusion and the effect on the vascular resistance, motility and electrical activity of the preparation observed. We have found toxic effects, if any, to be usually upon the motor activity, and the action of one PVC, used early in our perfusion work, on the otherwise normal motility of a stomach-duodenum preparation, is shown in Figure 8.

Circuit Fittings

Cannulae

The choice of cannula depends very much on the vessels selected and should be chosen or designed with each individual preparation in mind. There are three broad categories. Firstly those which are constructed for a particular size of vessel, or to lie at a particular angle to the preparation. These are usually best made from stainless steel and should have two rims to prevent slipping when tied into the vessel. Such a cannula may incorporate a side-arm for the measurement of pressure.

Secondly, the ordinary straight plastic connectors of suitable size are extremely useful and easy to manipulate. Thirdly, for retrograde cannulation of the aorta, and for cannulation of other vessels to bleed the animal prior to perfusion, a length of semi-rigid PVC tubing will be found ideal. A little sterile paraffin will ease its passage if the vessel is rather small, and avoid stripping of the intima.

Taps and Connectors

A tap is required in the arterial line for the injection of drugs, sampling of blood and measurement of pressure. Ideally this should be as close to the preparation as possible, and if a segment of aorta is included, then the top end of this provides the best site. A small

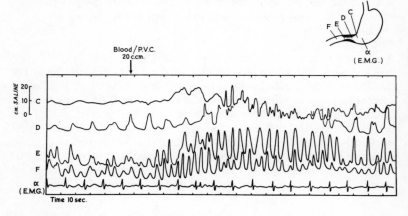

Fig. 8 Open tip tubes in the stomach and duodenum recorded normal motor activity, left hand side of trace. Intra-arterial injection of 20 ml of blood exposed to PVC tubing for two hours stimulated marked increase in gastric and duodenal motility.

disposable plastic stopcock is easily held in place here with a stout ligature. If this site is not available, then stainless steel fittings, of the same internal diameter as the tubing, may be used. They should have rimmed ends to ensure a snug fit inside the tubing (Figure 9). The placement of taps will depend upon the individual requirements. Connectors may also need to be used particularly if the circuit is complex or single lines need to be split or diverted. Plastic connectors are readily available for use in cardiovascular surgery; again the internal diameter should be the same as that of the tubing, the end barbed, and the inside highly polished to minimise trauma to the blood. Y or T shaped connectors should conform to the same

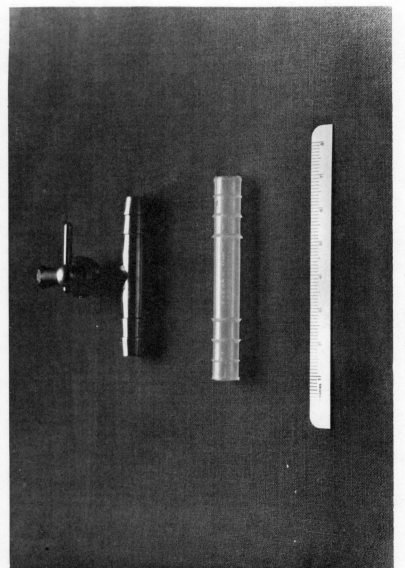

Fig. 9 Tap and Connector

standards and in the former the arm of the Y should not present too wide an angle to the flow of blood.

Prevention of Leakage

During the assembly of the circuit it is important that all points of connection are tight, particularly on the arterial side where pressure is high. Failure to ensure this may lead to troublesome leakage of blood, or sometimes, under certain conditions, a Venturi effect which will cause air to be drawn into the system. This is avoided first of all by the use of tubing and rimmed connections of matched size which fit snugly together. If however for some reason the tubing requires to be tightened down on to a somewhat smaller fitting, then this can be done using soft 20-gauge copper wire or one of the self locking nylon ties that are available.

The Venous Reservoir

This has always presented a problem in perfusion work for a number of reasons. It must accommodate from 100 cc to over a litre of blood, depending upon how much is added to or removed from the circuit during the course of an experiment. It may need to be raised or lowered both to control the level of blood in the oxygenator, and to facilitate drainage from the preparation. Ideally air should be excluded and the blood must not be allowed to stagnate. The position of the inlet and outlet should therefore be such as to encourage mixing.

One solution to these problems is offered here and makes use of collapsible plastic packs of intravenous fluids. These usually have a single outlet at the bottom, and if combined with a stainless steel fitting that permits entry of blood via a centre channel and exit via a concentric outer channel, a functional reservoir is obtained (Figure 10). It may then be suspended from an arm, the height of which is variable with respect to the oxygenator.

Cleaning and Care of the Apparatus

Greatest attention must be paid to cleaning the apparatus. The technique we recommend is as follows. It will be seen that sterilising is not essential for most short-term studies.

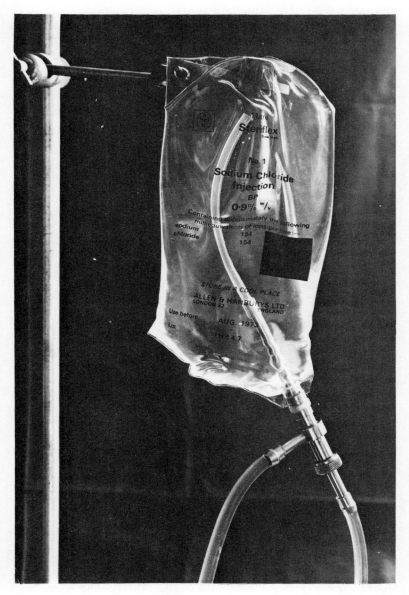

Fig. 10 Venous reservoir.

1. Strip down all apparatus
2. Discard disposable elements
3. Wash and scrub all re-usable apparatus (pumps etc.) in Teepol. Make sure all blood residues are removed
4. Soak in hydrogen peroxide overnight
5. Wash in running tap water
6. Wash in distilled water
7. Dry for 2 hours in air
8. Assemble all apparatus and make circuit
9. Recirculate distilled water   (2 litres) $\frac{3}{4}$ hr
10. Recirculate saline   (2 litres) $\frac{3}{4}$ hr
11. Recirculate tyrode   (1 litre) $\frac{1}{2}$ hr

The apparatus is now ready for priming.

If perfusion is to be carried out using undiluted blood the last step in this procedure may be omitted and the circuit primed after discarding the saline wash.

We have found that bacterial contamination may be a problem in those parts of the apparatus which are not disposable. *Pseudomonas pyocyanaeus* and *E. coli* have been cultured on occasions and it is not possible to remove such contaminants by the ordinary washing process. (Sterilisation with ethylene oxide is necessary in such circumstances.) It is important to realise that this may occur and swabs should be taken from the apparatus at intervals. The routine use of antibiotics added to the perfusion should help to reduce this problem.

References

Bjork, V.O. (1948) Brain perfusions in dogs with artificially oxygenated blood. *Acta. Chir. Scand.* **96,** Suppl. 137.

Brodie, T.G. (1903) The perfusion of surviving organs. *J. Physiol.* **29,** 266.

Duke, H.N., Vane, J.R. (1968) An adverse effect of PVC used in extra-corporeal circulation. *Lancet* **ii,** 21.

Giron, F., Birtwell, W.C., Soroff, H.S. and Deterling, R.A. (1966) Haemodynamic effects of pulsatile and non-pulsatile flow. *Arch. Surg.* **93,** 802.

Guess, W.L. and Stetson, J.B. (1968) Tissue reactions to organotin stabilised PVC catheters. *J. Am. Med. Ass.* **204,** 580.

Hooker, D.R. (1910) A study of the isolated kidney. The influence of pulse pressure on renal function. *Am. J. Physiol.* **27,** 24.

Jablonski, P., Douglas, M.C., Gordon, E., Owen, J.A. and Watts, J.McK. (1971) Studies on the isolated perfused pig liver. *Brit. J. Surgery* **58**, 129.

Jacobs, L.A., Klopp, E.M., Seamone, W., Topaz, S.R. and Gott, V.L. (1969) Improved organ function during cardiac by-pass with a roller pump modified to deliver pulsatile flow. *J. Thor. and Cardiovasc. Surg.* **58**, 703.

Kelman, G.R. and Nunn, J.F. (1966) Nomograms for correction of blood PO_2, PCO_2, pH and base excess for time and temperature. *J. Appl. Physiol.* **21**, 454.

Lee, W.H., Krummaar, D., Derry, G., Sachs, D., Lawrence, S.M., Clowes, G.H.A. and Maloney, J.F. (1961) Comparison of the effects of membrane and non-membrane oxygenators on the biochemical and biophysical characteristics of blood. *Surg. Forum* **12**, 200.

Little, K. and Parkhouse, J. (1962) Tissue reactions to polymers. *Lancet* **ii**, 857.

Melrose, D.G., Bramson, M.L., Osborn, J.J. and Gerbode, F. (1958) The membrane oxygenator: some aspects of oxygen and carbon dioxide transport across polythene film. *Lancet* **i**, 1050.

Miller, B.J., Gibbon, J.M.Jnr. and Gibbon, M.H. (1951) Recent advances in the development of a mechanical heart and lung apparatus. *Ann. Surg.* **1** (34), 694.

Parsons, R.J. and McMaster, P.D. (1938) Effect of pulse upon formation and flow of lymph. *J. Exp. Med.* **68**, 377.

Shepherd, R.B. and Kirklin, J.W. (1969) Relation of pulsatile flow to oxygen consumption and other variables during cardiopulmonary by-pass. *J. Thor. and Cardiovasc. Surg.* **58**, 694.

Trinkel, J.K., Helton, N.E., Bryant, L.R. and Wood, R.C. (1968) Metabolic comparison of pulsatile and mean flow for cardiopulmonary by-pass. *Circulation* **38**, Suppl. VI, 196.

Trinkel, J.K., Helton, N.E., Bryant, L.R. and Griffin, W.O. (1971) Pulsatile cardiopulmonary by-pass – clinical evaluation. *Surgery* **68**, 1074.

CHAPTER SIX

Perfusion Fluid and Choice of Flow Rate

Perfusion Fluid

The ideal perfusate should closely resemble normal whole animal blood. It should have a high O_2 carrying capacity, and colloid osmotic pressure and ionic composition comparable to the intact animal. Many workers have found it has been necessary to use pooled homologous blood owing to the low blood volume supplied by the donor animal. The large blood volume of the greyhound permits the use of autologous blood, which undoubtedly produces improved results. Priming of the circuit before perfusion with a non-sanguineous fluid inevitably results in some admixture of whole blood and primer. In liver perfusion it is our practice to use blood perfusate at a reduced haematocrit.

In practice the perfusate used is autologous blood diluted to a greater or lesser degree depending on certain technical requirements. The composition of the primer is adjusted to produce a perfusate similar to whole blood with respect to electrolyte and protein concentration. In this way selected haematocrit values can be obtained whilst electrolyte and protein concentrations remain within normal limits.

In the greyhound liver, the use of the animal's whole blood (haematocrit 65–70) is associated with the early onset of increased vascular resistance and failure of the perfused organ. With blood at such a high haematocrit, perfusion pressures are high for a given flow rate. This tends to produce congestive changes, which can be shown to resolve if the haematocrit is immediately lowered. The resistance to flow in a tube is proportional to the viscosity. Above values of 45–50, viscosity increases at a progressively greater rate with gradual haematocrit increments. Below this value, the relationship of viscosity to haematocrit is nearly linear. It is our experience that liver perfusion progresses more satisfactorily at perfusate haematocrit values of 30–40.

In contrast, stomach, gastro-oesophageal and duodenal preparations when perfused with whole blood behave in a stable and predictable way relatively free from congestion or oedema for a 4–5 hour period. The difference may partly reflect the marked sensitivity of the canine liver towards developing outflow block, but trauma to the perfusing blood may also be a factor.

The problem of trauma to elements of the blood is common to all pump oxygenator systems. Studies monitoring haemolysis of blood circulated in perfusion systems *in vitro* show a steady rise in free haemoglobin. This is related to flow rate, duration of perfusion and haematocrit (Cahill and Kolff, 1959; Ferkers and Kirkland, 1958). Red cell trauma is accompanied by trauma to other elements, particularly platelets. Recirculation experiments demonstrate a gradual fall in platelet count. This is associated with release of thromboplastins and activation of plasminogen. The blood may show increased coagulability with formation of microthrombi (Gans *et al*, 1962). Canine red cells are less resistant to trauma than those of most other species including man. Evidence that free haemoglobin may directly damage organs (Miller and McDonald, 1951) adds an additional rationale for minimising the red cell destruction in perfusion work. Where perfusion flow rate is high (e.g. 500–700 ml/min) as in the liver, haemolysis can be reduced by lowering the haematocrit.

In our view the use of autologous red cells is an essential part of canine organ perfusion technique. The large blood volume of the greyhound avoids the necessity for homologous red cell supplements, essential for sanguineous rat organ perfusions. Andrews *et al* (1955) showed that early outflow block occurred when homologous blood was used, despite careful crossmatching. Eiseman *et al* (1963) supported this conclusion and showed in pigs that addition of unmatched homologous blood to a liver perfusion circuit, where inflow was by gravity, caused a marked fall in total hepatic blood flow.

Both heparin and purified Malayan pit viper venom (Arvin) have proved satisfactory as anticoagulants. Citrate is not suitable as it reduces the pH of the perfusing medium and leads to a fall in the calcium concentration.

Malayan pit viper venom, which lowers the blood fibrinogen level, must be given to the dog for a period of 2 days before perfusion. Bleeding during surgery is not a problem and the elimination of fibrin aggregates may improve the quality of the perfused organ.

Heparin is more convenient. It is readily available, anticoagulation is effective and its onset rapid. However, interaction with other agents such as steroids may render its use unsuitable for a particular experiment and it is known to reduce gastric acid secretion. Heparin is given in a dose of 2–4 mg/kg body weight. Half this dose is added to the priming fluid in the reservoir and half is given intravenously just before the circuit is primed with autologous blood. The half life of heparin is about 120 minutes and during perfusion further additions are made. Where diluted whole blood is used, the ionic composition of the perfusate is maintained by the use of physiological solution adjusted to resemble intact greyhound serum. Sodium and chloride concentrations in intact greyhound plasma are higher than in the human. A Krebs solution modified to a comparable ionic composition is used.

NaCl	25·6g
NaHCO$_3$	8·82 g
KHCO$_3$	1·6 g
CaCl$_2$	0·4 g
MgCl$_2$	0·8 g
NaH$_2$PO$_4$	4·0 g
Glucose	2·0 g
Distilled water (sterilised)	4,000 ml

This solution has the following composition:

Sodium	155 mEq/l
Chloride	115 mEq/l
Potassium	4 mEq/l
Bicarbonate	26 mEq/l
Calcium	10 mg/100 ml
Glucose	50 mg/100 ml

Most workers recommend that low molecular weight dextran, albumin or similar colloid preparations should be added to the perfusate, but objective evidence of their efficacy in preventing oedema has been lacking. In dog liver, Shoemaker (1960) mentions that dilution of the perfusate leads to oedema, whilst histological evidence suggested that perfusion of the pig liver with Ringer lactate led to marked oedema which was improved by subsequent addition of low molecular weight dextran (Hobbs et al, 1968).

It is the impression in this department, that low perfusate protein levels are associated with visible oedema of the isolated perfused canine stomach. Measurement of the extracellular fluid space using C^{14} inulin shows high values in the canine liver when the protein concentration is low (Nicholls, 1972). Plasma albumin values greater than 3 g% seem satisfactory. Preparations of bovine albumin or expired human plasma protein fraction can be added to the perfusate, but perfusate electrolyte concentration, especially potassium should be monitored. Protein supplements are preferred to the use of low molecular weight dextran, since plasma protein estimations can be more easily performed.

References

Andrews, W.H.H., Hecker, R., Maegraith, B.G. and Ritchie, H.D. (1955) The action of adrenaline, L-noradrenaline, acetylcholine and other substances on the blood vessels of the perfused canine liver. *J. Physiol.* **128,** 413.

Cahill, J.J. and Kolff, W.J. (1959) Haemolysis caused by pumps in extracorporeal circuit. *J. Appl. Physiol.* **14,** 1039.

Eiseman, B., Knipe, P., Koh, Y., *et al.* (1963) Factors affecting hepatic vascular resistance in the perfused liver. *Ann. Surg.* **157,** 532.

Ferkers, E.W. and Kirkland, J.W. (1958) Studies of haemolysis with plastic sheet bubble oxygenator. *J. Thoracic Surg.* **36,** 23.

Gans, H., Lillehei, C.W. and Krivit, W. (1962) Problems in haemostasis during open heart surgery. II: On the hypercoagulability of the blood. *Ann. Surg.* **156,** 19.

Hobbs, K.E.F., Hunt, A.C., Palmer, D.B., Badrick, F.E., Morris, A.M., Mitra, S.K., Peacock, J.H., Immeman, E.J. and Riddell, A.G. (1968) Hypothermic low flow liver perfusion as a means of porcine hepatic storage for 6 hours. *Brit. J. Surg.* **55,** 696.

Miller, J.H. and McDonald, R.K. (1951) The effect of haemoglobin on renal function in the human. *J. Clin. Invest.* **30,** 1033.

Nicholls, R.J. (1972) Unpublished observations.

Shoemaker, W.C., Panico, F.G., Walker, W.F. and Elwyn, D.H. (1960) Perfusion of canine liver *in vivo. J. Appl. Physiol.* **15,** (4) 687.

Flow Rate

One of the chief assets of isolated organ perfusion is that at all times the flow of blood to the organ can be controlled. Changes in the preparation therefore can only be ascribed to a change in flow when this has deliberately been varied by the experimenter. In this system both flow and perfusing pressure are known. Much organ perfusion work especially in the liver has been done with portal venous flow provided by a gravity feed system from a reservoir at a known height above the preparation. During an isolated organ perfusion, vascular resistance sometimes changes spontaneously and, for a given head of pressure, flow will change. In a gravity feed system therefore the flow rate is not maintained steady. Bauer *et al* (1932) had to raise the height of their gravity feed to a very high level to maintain flow. Eiseman (1963) showed that in a fixed gravity system, flow in the isolated pig liver fell to 50% of initial values after 4 hours and a greater fall occurred in the dog. Not all workers have reported such flow changes; Van Wyk *et al* (1965) were able to maintain total hepatic blood flow for several hours in pig livers rendered totally ischaemic at room temperature for up to 3 hours before perfusion.

It is our practice to use calibrated pumps so that perfusion flow rate at all times is known. In the intestine where motility has been shown to alter blood flow (Sidky and Bean, 1958) a steady flow enhances the stability of the preparation and the reproducibility of some of its responses.

Under basal conditions the flow requirements of an organ on perfusion seem to differ little from those estimated from intact animal experiments.

Values of 25 ml/kg body wt/min for portal venous flow in the intact dog (Stewart *et al*, 1958) corresponding to 500 ml/min for a 20 kg dog, are only slightly higher than the portal venous flow used for our canine liver perfusion. Estimates of blood flow in stomach (35 ml/min/100 g), intestine (50 ml/min/100 g) and pancreas (80 ml/min/100 g) for the intact dog (Grim, 1963) are a little higher than the flow rates used in perfusions of these organs in the isolated situation.

The most easily monitored criterion of adequate perfusion flow rate is that of oxygen uptake by the preparation. Where flow is adjusted to produce an arteriovenous oxygen saturation difference of 30% the flow is deemed satisfactory (Ritchie *et al*, 1962). Using this as a baseline we have found that satisfactory perfusions are obtained with the canine stomach at 40 ml per minute (10–20 ml/min/100 g), the pancreas at 25 ml per minute (20–40 ml/min/100 g) and the liver at 500–600 ml per minute (60–100 ml/min/100 g).

There is good anatomical (Barlow, 1951) and functional evidence (Sherman and Newman, 1954) that extensive sub-mucosal arteriovenous shunts exist in the stomach and small intestine. Measurement of the venous oxygen saturation in perfused preparations may be misleading where shunting is going on. If some arterial blood passes unchanged to the venous side of the preparation, the venous oxygen saturation may rise by 5–10% giving values of 80%. This cannot in these circumstances be accepted as indicating adequate perfusion of the whole organ. Xenon studies with our preparation of the stomach suggest that arteriovenous shunts are open in at least half the preparations and that as much as one fifth of the total flow may on occasion pass through them.

Arterial pressure in all isolated preparations is low, usually 60 mm Hg and seldom more than 100 mm Hg. In spite of this, perfusion as judged by other criteria is adequate, and we believe it to reflect the complete autonomic denervation of the organ, and the lack of circulating catecholamines with consequent loss of vascular tone. Pressure therefore is an unreliable guide to the adequacy of perfusion and should be used only as an indication of changes in vascular resistance which may for example be induced in all these preparations by the administration of vaso-active drugs.

Overperfusion is associated with certain recognisable changes in the preparation and should be corrected before irreversible damage has occurred. Perfusion pressure will be high and 80 mm Hg is regarded as abnormal in the absence of any mechanical obstruction to flow such as may occur with kinking of a line or the formation of clot due to inadequate heparinisation. The venous oxygen saturation will also be high, and a value of more than 80% suggests an excess of flow for the metabolic needs of the organ. Oedema formation is increased. In the liver ascites pours from the surface, its weight increases, and measurements of red cell mass and tissue extracellular water show an associated rise. The liver reacts to overperfusion by an increase in its vascular resistance and portal venous pressure will show a gradual rise. In other preparations visible oedema will appear; around the pancreas, in the omentum and in the sub-mucosa of the stomach, and as a transudate into the gastric lumen. Small petechial haemorrhages will appear and sometimes frank haematomata. The gastric secretion may become tinged with blood as may the bile and lymph from the liver.

Underperfusion is not such a serious problem, many of these organs exhibiting a remarkable tolerance to reductions in flow that lead to venous oxygen saturations of 20% or less. The canine liver is an exception being very sensitive to ischaemia and reacting to it with the development of acidosis, release of intracellular potassium and venous outflow block. The stomach on the other hand, apart from slowing of the gastric pace-setter potential, continues to exhibit motility and to secrete acid, with flow reduced to one quarter of normal.

Flow in a perfused organ therefore depends upon the pump, and the control of the pump is in the hands of the experimenter. During the initial stages it is safer to underperfuse the preparation as it is more likely to tolerate this without the appearance of irreversible damage. Once the period of recovery has passed, all these preparations will be found to exhibit very stable conditions of flow and pressure unless deliberate changes are made to the pump output, or vaso-active drugs are administered to the preparation.

We have confirmed the macroscopic adequacy of perfusion by angiography and radiographs will be found in the chapters on individual organs. We have also used a radioactive Xenon 133 washout technique according to the method described by Thorburn *et al* (1963) for the study of intrarenal blood flow to ascertain that the distribution of blood to the various tissue compartments of a perfused organ is adequate. At the present time our work with the canine stomach would suggest that there is no significant difference in total blood flow under basal conditions between the intact, and the isolated perfused stomach. Moreover its distribution to mucosa and muscle appears to be the same in both situations.

The presence of functioning sub-mucosal shunts in the isolated preparation has also been demonstrated using this technique and they would appear to play an important rôle in the control of blood flow to the mucosa.

References

Barlow, T.E. (1951) Arteriovenous anastomoses in the human stomach. *J. Anat.* **85**, 1.

Bauer, W., Dale, H.H., Poulsson, L.T. and Richards, D.W. (1932) The control of circulation through the liver. *J. Physiol.* **74**, 343.

Eiseman, B., Knipe, P., and Koh, Y. (1963) Factors affecting hepatic vascular resistance in the perfused liver. *Ann. Surg.* **157**, 532.

Grim, E. (1963) *Handbook of Physiology.* Volume 2 *Circulation*, 1439.

Ritchie, H.D., Freeman, M.A.R., Shaw, D., and Toner, J. (1962) The value of rapid blood oxygen saturation determinations during heart-lung by-pass experiments. *J. Roy. Coll. Surg. Ed.* **7,** 295.

Sherman, J.L.Jr. and Newman, S. (1954) Functioning arteriovenous anastomoses in the stomach and duodenum. *Amer. J. Physiol.* **179,** 279.

Sidky, M. and Bean, J.W. (1958) The influence of rhythmic and tonic contraction of intestinal muscle on blood flow and blood reservoir capacity in dog intestine. *Am. J. Physiol.* **193,** 386.

Stewart, J.D., Stephens, J.G., Leslie, M.B., Portin, B.A. and Schenk, W.G. (1958) Portal haemodynamics under varying experimental conditions. *Ann. Surg.* **147,** 868.

Thorburn, G.D., Kopald, H.H., Herd, J.A., Hollenberg, M., O'Morchoe, C.C.C. and Barger, A.C. (1963) Intrarenal distribution of nutrient blood flow determined with Krypton 85 in the un-anaesthetised dog. *Circ. Res.* **13,** 290.

Van Wyk, J., Leim, D.S. and Eiseman, B. (1965) Function of cadaver liver. *Surgery* **58,** 120.

CHAPTER SEVEN

Monitoring

It has already been made clear that the great advantage of the isolated preparation is that intrinsic physiological responses can be studied. On the other hand, the fact that it is isolated means that there is disruption of its extrinsic homeostatic mechanisms. The extent of this disruption is difficult to determine because of our lack of knowledge of basic physiological control mechanisms. The preparation however has to be maintained in as physiological a condition as possible. This can only be done in relation to known physiological parameters. Some of the parameters we have monitored are to be found in the circulating perfusate, and their values will depend to a certain extent on the perfusate's dilution and the type of diluent. Others which we believe should be routinely studied are listed below. All will be discussed individually.

1. Blood flow
2. Arterial and venous pressures
3. Temperature
4. Haemolysis
5. Haematocrit
6. Arterial and venous pH
7. Blood gases
8. Blood biochemistry
   (a) Electrolytes
   (b) Plasma proteins
   (c) Blood sugars
9. Blood loss from the preparation

Blood Flow

This has already been dealt with in an earlier section. It may crudely be regarded as being satisfactory if the preparation looks well perfused as judged by colour, if the venous oxygen saturation lies between 55–70% and in the hollow viscus preparation, if it appears to contract well. In most perfusions a constant outflow pump is used and it is unnecessary to monitor blood flow as the pump setting can be altered to give any desired output. Some stomach perfusions have been performed using a pulsatile pump which does not give a constant output. Blood flow in these perfusions is continuously monitored using an electromagnetic flow meter inserted into the arterial line. Recommended blood flow values for specific perfusions are given in the relevant sections.

Blood Pressure

(1) Arterial

In stomach perfusions where the arterial cannula is placed in a cuff of aorta the arterial pressure at the time the organ is switched on to perfusion slowly rises to between 50 and 80 mm which is the normal perfusion pressure. This may be regarded as being very low when compared with a normal systolic pressure of the greyhound (about 180 mm Hg). If flow however is adjudged to be adequate with regard to the above criteria, then the difference in pressures should be due to a fall in peripheral resistance. This may result from reduced sympathetic stimulus associated with a fall in circulating catecholamines and sympathetic denervation.

In the liver both portal venous and hepatic arterial blood pressures are monitored. As in the stomach, the flow rate is constant so a rise in pressure indicates an increase in the intrahepatic resistance. The beginning of perfusion is often associated with a rise in portal venous and hepatic arterial pressures and this is thought to be associated with a catecholamine response to bleeding for priming. After an initial period the portal venous pressure should settle at 10 cm blood and the hepatic arterial pressure at 80–100 mm Hg. A rise in portal venous pressure in the course of a perfusion generally indicates deterioration of the preparation, which is most likely due to the syndrome of 'venous outflow block'.

The important point to realise about the perfusion pressure is that as long as flow is judged to be satisfactory the pressure is not critical.

(2) Venous

Venous pressure and venous return are monitored by a side-arm on the venous line. Continuous measurement can be obtained by attaching the electromagnetic flow meter to the venous line.

With a constant arterial inflow, a fall in venous return is due either to haemorrhage from the preparation, venous outflow block or obstruction of the venous cannula. The former is easily recognised but venous obstruction, although relatively easy to detect in hollow viscus perfusion with visible venous engorgement, is more difficult to recognise in hepatic perfusions. The cause of obstruction is usually torsion of the venous pedicle.

The ideal venous pressure is 0 to −1 cm blood. A negative pressure is obtained by arranging that the venous reservoir and oxygenator lie below the level of the perfusion chamber. Care must be taken to avoid too great a negative pressure, otherwise the venous radicle undergoes the phenomenon known as 'venous flutter'. In such cases, the venous reservoir is too far below the venous pedicle, the intervening column of blood acts as a syphon, produces an increased negative pressure and collapse of the vein. This blocks the venous return, abolishes the syphonage effect and the vein reopens. This sequence of events results in intermittent periods of venous drainage.

A high venous pressure will alter the fluid dynamics at a capillary level and tend to produce tissue oedema. Xenon clearance measurements, which can be taken as a measure of capillary blood flow, show that a raised venous pressure produces a fall in capillary blood flow.

At venous pressure values of 0 to −5 cm blood, good capillary blood flow is obtained and the 'flutter' effect is negligible.

Temperature

Preparations are maintained at a temperature of 37°C. This is measured with either an electrical thermometer attached to the arterial line or in the case of liver perfusion by inserting a needle thermocouple directly into a liver lobule.

A high humidity is obtained by covering all preparations with a sheet of polythene and if possible enclosing it in a chamber.

Haemolysis

The amount of free plasma haemoglobin is taken as an indication of the degree of haemolysis. It is measured spectrophotometrically and expressed in milligrams of free haemoglobin per 100 ml of blood. It is impossible to lay down definite values for acceptable haemolysis rates – except to say that the rise in plasma haemoglobin should be as little as possible. Haemolysis is produced by blood damage chiefly caused by the pump, oxygenator and the perfusion tubing, and will vary according to the types of apparatus used.

Haemolysis rates are meaningless when monitored during a liver perfusion because the free haemoglobin is cleared from the plasma by the liver and as such the plasma values are falsely low. Separate experiments using a liverless circuit should be performed.

Haematocrit

The choice of a suitable packed cell volume at which to perfuse has been dealt with earlier in Chapter 6. In essence, the packed cell volume can be high in perfusions where the blood flow is small, e.g. stomach, but needs to be low where flows are high, e.g. liver. Hence, the haematocrit is more critical in hepatic perfusion and at least one value should be obtained at the start of each experiment. This is not absolutely necessary in the hollow viscus perfusions. Serial haematocrit readings show a slight rise over the course of a three-hour perfusion. This is probably due to evaporation and to the loss of other biological fluids, e.g. lymph, exocrine secretion, from the preparation.

Arterial and Venous pH

In man the pH of blood is maintained within a narrow physiological range. Immediate compensation for changes in hydrogen and bi-carbonate ion concentration is provided by the blood buffers. Buffer concentration is then later replenished by renal and pulmonary excretion of the unwanted ion. In isolated organ perfusion the latter mechanism is absent and maintenance of a physiological pH range is dependent on the blood buffers. This is not always adequate and it is sometimes necessary to correct for changes in blood pH. (Figure 13)

Serial pH readings have been taken in an attempt to determine the extent of this disturbance, and the efficacy of its correction by the addition of bicarbonate. Because the oxygenator is exposed to such a high concentration of oxygen (see later) any disturbance is taken as being metabolic in nature and not due to inefficient oxygenation.

Arterial pH

The 'physiological' range is taken to be 7·35–7·45. In a series of 43 isolated stomach perfusions 164 pH readings were taken. 67% of these were within the normal range. The remaining 33% were below a pH of 7·35. These low values were corrected by the addition of 8·4% solution of sodium bicarbonate. Of the 43 perfusions there were 26 in which bicarbonate was added. In these the initial mean pH was 7·34 ± 0·05. An average of 8·5 mEq of bicarbonate was added to each of these perfusions, which increased the mean pH to 7·41 ± 0·05. The quantities needed were calculated using a Siggaard-Andersen nomogram or a blood gas calculator. If the pH, pCO_2 and haemoglobin are known, then the concentration of HCO_3 and CO_2 in the plasma can be calculated. An analysis of all the experiments showed that the mean pH during the first hour was 7·38 ± 0·09, during the second 7·30 ± 0·06 and during the third 7·40 ± 0·07.

It will be seen from these results that it is common for there to be a mild metabolic acidosis. This needs correction with sodium bicarbonate and it is most likely to occur within the first hour of perfusion. An acidosis within the first hour of perfusion is common in the liver, stomach, oesophagus, pancreas and biliary perfusions. It is particularly common in the secretin stimulated pancreas which is actively clearing bicarbonate from the perfusate.

Venous pH

Changes occur *pari passu* with changes in the arterial pH and are generally 0·02 pH unit below the arterial value. The one exception is in the acid secreting stomach where there is an arterial/venous pH reversal.

Blood Gases

(1) Arterial pO_2 and oxygen saturation.

The oxygenator is exposed to a gas mixture containing 95% oxygen and 5% carbon dioxide, so with a partial pressure of oxygen ranging between 300–450 mm Hg 100% oxygen saturation is easily obtained. Prolonged exposure to 100% oxygen in man is known to be toxic. This is not thought to be the case in isolated organ perfusion. No noticeable differences have been observed in the performance of the isolated organ when high and low oxygen percentages have been used.

(2) Venous pO_2 and oxygen saturation

The importance of the relationship of blood flow and venous oxygen saturation has already been discussed.

Blood Biochemistry

Electrolytes, blood glucose and plasma proteins should be measured and may be taken as an indication of the ionic, metabolic and colloid status of the perfusate. The importance of the type and quantity of the diluent in the perfusate has already been stressed but further more specific comments will be made in each section.

(a) Electrolytes

I. Sodium and chloride
In all preparations, provided the diluent has a similar sodium chloride content to greyhound plasma, e.g. Tyrode's solution or normal saline, then levels within the normal range are maintained over a three-hour period. However, there appears to be a gradual rise in concentration over this period which, if taken in conjunction with the rising packed cell volume, indicates haemoconcentration.

II. Potassium
In hollow viscus perfusions the plasma potassium levels are found to remain within normal limits and constant over a period of three hours. In liver perfusion plasma potassium values seem to follow a set pattern. There is an initial increase due to the loss of potassium from the liver which occurs in the first 10 minutes. Over the next 60 minutes the plasma potassium falls as the liver takes up potassium. Thereafter, the potassium levels remain steady.

Plasma potassium changes have not been found to be a useful guide as to the degree of haemolysis occurring.

III. Bicarbonate
Although strictly an electrolyte, this ion is of more importance in the control of blood pH. The levels are usually initially low in

association with a metabolic acidosis and need correction by adding bicarbonate. This has already been discussed.

IV. Calcium

Control of calcium levels is of greatest importance in the hollow viscus perfusions where myoelectrical activity is being recorded. Earlier stomach perfusion used a Krebs/Ringer/bicarbonate solution as a diluent and in these preparations it was found that calcium levels fell steadily during a 3-hour perfusion. One of the problems was that before being added to the blood the calcium and bicarbonate content of the diluent tended to precipitate as calcium carbonate. Since this has been abandoned and small quantities of normal saline have been substituted as a primer the calcium levels remain constant. The values are slightly lower than in the normal greyhound, which is unavoidable because some dilution must occur.

(b) Blood Glucose

The blood glucose levels in stomach perfusions when no sugar was added to the circuit during perfusion showed a gradual fall, which was presumably due to the sugar being metabolised. It is now customary to add glucose regularly. A relatively constant level of blood sugar can be maintained if 200 mg of dextrose are added at 30-minute intervals.

In liver perfusion the blood glucose pattern differs from that seen in hollow viscus preparations. There is an initial increase in the blood sugar associated with a fall in liver glycogen content. This lasts for about 30 minutes and is followed by a slow decrease in blood glucose over the next hour as the liver takes up glucose. This is then followed by steady levels over the next 90 minutes. It is not therefore necessary to add glucose to the circuit in liver perfusion. There are enormous glycogen reserves which can maintain steady levels.

(c) Plasma Proteins

Oedema formation will result in poor organ function. The chief oedema preventing factor is the colloid osmotic pressure of the perfusate. It is therefore important to maintain the plasma protein concentration as near normal as possible.

The total plasma protein concentration in the stomach perfusions where little dilution of the perfusate has occurred is less than normal but the values remain constant throughout the perfusion. Subjectively, in perfusions where little dilution has occurred the preparations appear to be less oedematous. Therefore if the dilution volume is small it would seem unnecessary to add colloids.

In the liver, however, where a low packed cell volume is used, it is necessary to add colloid to maintain an effective osmotic pressure. This has been done by using discarded human plasma as a diluent. In this way it is possible to maintain a steady plasma protein concentration above 4 grams %. If plasma is not available then Rheomacrodex (0·6%) and Macrodex (0·4%) can be used.

Loss of Blood and other fluids

Some blood loss is unavoidable from all preparations. A loss of 50–100 ml/blood/hour is acceptable. Measurements of loss of lymph and exocrine secretion are not generally monitored except in experiments where they are of especial interest. These will be mentioned in the relevant chapters in Part 2.

PART TWO

CHAPTER EIGHT

Liver

Perfusion of the Isolated Canine Liver

Introduction

In the twenties, advances in our knowledge of the liver came largely from the liver slice preparation developed by Warburg. However, with the discovery and later introduction of heparin, and development of new apparatus and materials, during the thirties, the isolated liver preparation became feasible, and has much to offer in the study of liver physiology.

The post-war introduction of plastic tubing, improvements in anaesthesia and advances in biochemical monitoring, helped the firm establishment of perfusion techniques.

With the development of satisfactory equipment for cardio-pulmonary by-pass, the problems of oxygenation and blood flow have been largely overcome. New pumps, oxygenators, disposable tubing, efficient heat exchangers and antibiotics have contributed to the great improvement in liver perfusion and preservation seen in the last twenty years.

The studies of Mautner and Pick (1915), are among the earliest where the isolated perfused liver was successfully used as a model in the investigation of a physiological problem. These workers drew attention to the occurrence of venous outflow block in the canine liver in response to histamine or peptone. The livers were perfused via the portal vein by gravity feed using either Ringer's solution or diluted blood as perfusate.

During the twenties, few sanguineous perfusions were undertaken. Baer and Roessler (1926) and Simonds and Brandes (1929) produced further evidence to suggest that histamine causes hepatic vein constriction in the dog. McLaughlin (1928) perfused the livers of several species with Ringer's solution but under conditions that in many experiments were unphysiological.

In 1928 Bauer, Dale et al developed a system for the sanguineous perfusion of the mammalian liver (Dale, 1929) and reported on their experience with perfusion of the livers of dog, cat and goat (Bauer, Dale et al, 1932). Both hepatic artery and portal vein were perfused, the latter by a fixed gravity system. They used a Hooker oxygenator, glass tubing with rubber connections, a Dale-Schuster pump for perfusion of the hepatic artery and a container for the liver in the form of a thermostatically controlled plethysmograph. The dog livers developed outflow block within one hour, but cat and goat livers survived longer. Chakravarti and Tripod (1940) used the same system but used the lungs of another dog in favour of the Hooker oxygenator.

These perfusions where portal vein flow rate diminished gradually owing to progressive increase in vascular resistance were criticised by Trowell (1942) who described a method of rat liver perfusion with Ringer's solution at a constant flow rate maintained by a pump.

In 1951, Brauer et al published a description of the sanguineous perfusion of the rat liver. This method has since been widely used as a model for biochemical and physiological studies.

Renewed interest in canine liver perfusion followed the description of an improved method of perfusion by Andrews (1953). Avoidance of any period of total ischaemia, the use of autologous blood and adjustable flow pumps improved the chances of survival. Subsequently the use of pump–oxygenator systems developed for extra-corporeal by-pass and adoption of PVC and silicone rubber tubing further improved the quality of perfused livers. The preparation became firmly established as a model for physiological studies (Andrews et al, 1955; Kestens et al, 1961; Shoemaker et al, 1960; Hardcastle and Ritchie, 1968).

In recent years other species have been used as donor animal, notably pig (Eiseman et al, 1964; Hickman et al, 1971; Hobbs et al, 1968), calf (Chapman et al, 1961; Condon et al, 1962) and baboon (Abouna et al, 1970).

The technical achievement of liver transplantation has in part stemmed from the development of the isolated perfused liver, and the demand for organ preservation continues to involve liver perfusion work.

The isolated perfused liver has also been developed as a means of extrahepatic support in selected patients with hepatic failure (Eiseman *et al*, 1964; Abouna *et al*, 1970; Hickman *et al*, 1971). Besides the great clinical interest generated by such work, the contribution to our knowledge of the basic activity and behaviour of the isolated liver preparation has been considerable.

Technique of Liver Perfusion

General Considerations
The greyhound liver is perfused via the portal vein and hepatic artery with autologous blood diluted with physiological solution to a haematocrit of 35. Blood leaving the liver via the hepatic veins drains by gravity to an Aga oxygenator and thence returns via a reservoir and heat exchanger to the portal vein and hepatic artery pumps. The temperature of the preparation is maintained at 38°C and total hepatic blood flow is adjusted to provide, under basal conditions, a fall in O_2 saturation of 30% from inflowing to hepatic venous blood.

In this system, the liver receives fully oxygenated blood from both hepatic artery and portal vein. Portal venous oxygen saturations of 60–70% can be obtained by the calculated admixture of oxygenated and hepatic venous blood. We have preferred to avoid the added problem of achieving lowered portal vein oxygen saturations and have obtained, as have other workers, satisfactory results using fully saturated blood.

One of the chief advantages that isolated organ perfusion offers as an experimental model is that at all times flow rate is accurately known and can be extrinsically controlled. The principle of gravity feed as a method of supplying the portal vein suffers from the disadvantage that flow changes with fluctuations in vascular resistance in the organ. We have avoided the use of such a system by the use of pumps where the flow can be maintained at a selected steady level.

The first hour of perfusion is a period when many of the parameters used to assess stability of the preparation are in a state of flux. During this time, portal pressure, initially high, gradually settles to a steady level. By the end of an hour, changes occurring in plasma potassium and glucose concentrations, seen at the start of perfusion, have largely resolved and bile flow, initially low, is likely to have increased to a steady level with, under basal conditions, a stable composition. Studies should therefore not be undertaken until this period has elapsed.

Apparatus and Perfusion Circuit

The portal vein is perfused by a non-pulsatile flow pump of screw type (Mono Pumps Ltd). Its priming capacity is 150 ml and it can be adjusted to deliver flows up to 1,000 ml/min.

An occlusive roller pump of the de Bakey type (Watson Marlow Pumps Ltd.) supplies the hepatic artery. Flows of 0–300 ml/min can be obtained with this model.

Silicone rubber or nylon cannulas are used. Tubing is renewed for each perfusion and lengths are joined by nylon connectors and Y-pieces. Metal taps are included in hepatic arterial, portal and hepatic venous lines.

The hepatic and portal venous lines terminate in specially constructed end pieces which are tied into the vessels cannulated. These possess a metal side-arm from which the lateral pressure in the lines can be measured.

The venous reservoir, made of Perspex, is graduated in 50 ml increments up to its total capacity of 2,000 ml. Blood from the oxygenator enters at a level corresponding to half the capacity and leaves along a cannula from its lowest part.

The heat exchanger, made of stainless steel, is interposed in the circuit between reservoir and pumps. It is circulated with water at 42°C from a thermostatically controlled heated water bath by a Stewart Turner electric pump delivering a flow of 2–3 l/min.

An oxygenator of the roller type similar to that in the Aga heart–lung machine is used in preference to the bubble oxygenator (Pulmopak) which produced excessive red cell trauma in earlier perfusions. The priming volume of 200–300 ml is satisfactory and its flow capacity of 1,000 ml/min adequate for the flows used.

The assembled circuit is shown in Figure 11.

Although only one is shown, blood leaves the liver by two cannulae inserted into the inferior vena cava, one above and the other below the liver. The two cannulae then join and the blood passes along a common venous return by gravity to the oxygenator. The blood is filmed over three rollers in a series and exposed to a gas mixture 95% O_2, 5% CO_2. It then flows to the reservoir. The blood is now drawn by the action of the pumps through the heat exchanger. The circuit is then divided. One line carries blood through the occlusive pump along a nylon cannula of external diameter 4 mm to the hepatic artery. The portal circulation is provided by the other line which passes through the constant flow pump via silicone rubber tubing to the portal vein. The priming volume of the circuit is about 800 ml.

The success of a liver perfusion depends greatly on the cleanliness of the apparatus. In the dog hepatic venous spasm rapidly ensues when the circuit has been inadequately washed clean. Foreign proteins and other vaso-active substances adherent to the non-disposable parts must be removed.

The perfusate used consists of a mixture of autologous blood and modified Krebs solution (see page 54).

The importance of using autologous blood will be discussed later. A haematocrit of 35, considerably lower than that of the intact greyhound (65–70), facilitates perfusion and leads to less red cell damage.

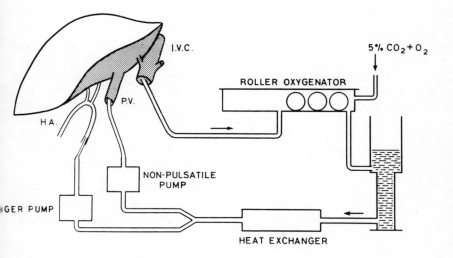

I.V.C.

5% $CO_2 + O_2$

ROLLER OXYGENATOR

P.V.

H A.

NON-PULSATILE PUMP

GER PUMP

HEAT EXCHANGER

Fig. 11 Isolated liver perfusion in the dog. Simplified diagram of the perfusion circuit.

The protein concentration of the perfusate may be adjusted by the addition of freeze-dried or other plasma protein preparations.

Heparin is used as anticoagulant in a dose of 2–4 mg/kg body weight. It should be given in divided doses, one to the reservoir initially primed with Krebs solution and one intravenously to the dog just before it is bled.

Water at 42°C is circulated through the heat exchanger at a rate of 2–3 l/min. An infra-red heater is mounted above the Aga oxygenator.

A rubber diaphragm in the portal venous line allows the insertion of a thermocouple probe and a similar probe may be inserted into the hepatic parenchyma. The reservoir stands three-quarters immersed in a constant temperature water bath. The preparation is covered with polythene sheeting to reduce heat and evaporation losses from its surface. Owing to the high perfusion flow rate per mass of tissue, the parenchymal temperature is well maintained by the perfusing blood; there is no need for warming of the organ directly by infra-red heaters.

The advantages of using the greyhound as the donor for isolated organ perfusion have already been indicated. The large volume of blood obtained from this species is of particular value in the isolated perfused canine liver preparation where perfusion flow rate and liver blood capacity are high.

The animal is not fed for 12 hours before perfusion.

Surgery

In the operation the portal vein, inferior vena cava above and below the liver and the hepatic artery are cannulated. The procedure described here is aimed at avoiding any period of total ischaemia or hypoxia. This is done by staggering the cannulation of portal vein and hepatic artery. Thus the liver is still perfused via the hepatic artery by the dog's own circulation, while the portal vein is cannulated. Perfusion via the portal vein is started and the hepatic artery finally cannulated. This procedure is done with the liver still lying within the dog's abdomen. If necessary, it can be removed at this stage.

The detailed account describes a satisfactory method for perfusing the liver. It is desirable that the operator develops a routine which suits him and does not alter. In this way mistakes are avoided and operating time kept to a minimum.

The surgical procedure will be considered in two parts. The first part describes the technique of perfusion where the liver is to remain within the carcass of the dog. The second describes the modifications and additional procedure necessary when it is required to remove the perfused liver from the dog to a specially constructed container.

The animal is induced with an intravenous injection of thiopentone in a dose of 20 mg/kg body weight. Once secured in the supine position on the table, an endotracheal tube is passed and the animal ventilated by an intermittent positive pressure respirator with 100% O_2 at a tidal volume of 300–400 ml. If the surgery is prolonged further intravenous thiopentone may be needed. The depth of anaesthesia should be carefully judged and should be sufficient to produce muscle relaxation.

In Situ Perfusion Bilateral inguinal incisions are made and the femoral vessels dissected out. Both femoral arteries are cannulated with No. 4 Portex nylon cannulae primed with heparinised saline and whose distal clamped ends are led into the reservoir. At a later stage these serve to bleed the dog and prime the circuit. A cannula for intravenous infusion of Krebs solution is inserted into the left femoral vein. During exsanguination, the infusion helps to maintain the blood pressure and improves the yield of perfusate.

A mid-line incision from xiphisternum to pubis is made and the peritoneal cavity opened. The wound is retracted by blunt hooks attached by cord to the sides of the table. The abdominal contents are carefully inspected.

The duodenum is held out of the wound by the assistant. This draws out the duodenal mesentery with the head of the pancreas between its two leaves, revealing in its base the superior mesenteric vein running towards the liver.

The peritoneum covering the superior mesenteric vein just caudal to its confluence with the splenic vein is incised and dissected from the vein wall. Two threads are passed behind the vessel and their ends secured with artery forceps. Any constriction of the vein by tension of the threads will diminish hepatic blood flow and must be avoided.

The pylorus and first part of the duodenum are now drawn down and to the left. This displays the structures within the free fold of the lesser omentum. The superior pancreatico-duodenal vein is identified and a thread passed around it. Further threads are passed around the gastro-duodenal artery and surrounding tissue, potentially isolating the structures supplied by the vessel.

A thread passed round the hepatic artery and held by forceps serves to enable the easy identification of the artery later in the procedure. At this stage the common bile duct is cannulated with a polyvinyl Portex No. 3 cannula and bile is allowed to flow freely. The cystic duct is carefully dissected out and tied off with a thread ligature.

The dog's lesser omentum is vascular and troublesome bleeding occurs unless it is divided between clamps and tied. The left gastric vessels are sought and ligated. A finger can now easily be hooked around the abdominal oesophagus and the whole stomach drawn down. Crushing clamps are applied to the oesophagus at the cardia and the gut is divided between them. It is now possible to reflect the stomach caudally and by this manoeuvre display the splenic vein. The peritoneum is divided over the splenic vein about 1 cm from its confluence with the superior mesenteric vein. At this point a thread tie is passed around the splenic vein to the liver side of entry of the inferior pancreatico-duodenal vein.

The abdominal dissection is complete.

The right femoral vein is cannulated centrally by one limb of the clamped venous return line. The tip of this wide-bore cannula is passed to lie just below the level of entry of the lowest hepatic vein into the inferior vena cava.

The dog is heparinised with a dose of 2–4 mg/kg body wt, half of which is given intravenously via the exposed left femoral vein, and the other half added to the reservoir.

After a short period to allow for heparinisation, the clamps on the femoral artery cannulae are released, the IV infusion accelerated and 500 ml of arterial blood are bled into the reservoir and the clamps re-applied. This acute blood loss causes the spleen to contract. The portal vein pump is switched on and the circuit primed with sanguineous perfusate. A clamp is applied to the portal venous line and the pump once again is switched off. The circuit is now ready.

A clamp now applied to the superior mesenteric artery reduces blood loss to the splanchnic bed. The superior mesenteric vein is tied distally, cutting off most of the portal flow to the liver. Drawing gently upward on the centrally placed thread to prevent back-bleeding, the portal venous cannula tip is introduced through a venotomy and tied firmly in place.

Clamps on the portal venous and hepatic venous lines in the femoral vein are released and perfusion started by switching on the portal venous pump. The animal is bled further into the reservoir by unclamping once again the femoral arterial cannulae.

Over the next 10 minutes, the portal flow is gradually increased from a starting value of 200 ml/min to the definitive selected value. By this time the reservoir should contain about 1–2 l of blood, the total volume of the circuit being about 3 l.

Two remaining surgical manoeuvres are required. The first is the isolation of the liver from its connections at the hilum with other organs; the second is the cannulation of the suprahepatic inferior vena cava.

The liver is isolated from all other organs draining into the portal system downstream from the perfusing cannula. The threads on the superior mesenteric vein and splenic vein are tied and the veins divided, thus excluding the liver from any remaining connection with the animal's portal system. The remaining structures in the free fold of the lesser omentum are divided between ties and the hepatic artery divided at its origin from the coeliac axis. With the gentle separation of any remaining non-vascular connections between pancreas and portal vein, the hilar structures become separated from all their *in vivo* connections. Isolation of the liver is complete within a few minutes of the onset of perfusion and the loss of perfusate into non-hepatic structures is minimal.

Attention is turned to the cannulation of the vena cava above the liver.

A mid-line incision is made from suprasternal notch to xiphisternum and the sternum is split longitudinally. On opening the chest, the suprahepatic inferior vena cava is identified and two threads passed round it. The tip of the second limb of the venous drainage cannula is brought to lie conveniently alongside the vessel. A venotomy is made, the cannula introduced and tied firmly in place and its clamp released permitting suprahepatic drainage of hepatic venous blood. During this procedure care must be taken to avoid air entering the vena cava. Gentle traction on the thread nearest the liver should produce complete temporary obstruction, preventing any air from getting in.

At this stage the liver is being perfused via the portal vein at a flow rate of 300–400 ml/min while hepatic venous blood drains freely along both supra- and infra-hepatic inferior vena cava cannulae to the oxygenator.

The hepatic arterial cannula is primed and the vessel easily identified by its previously placed surrounding ligature. After cannulation, flow is started by switching on the occlusive finger pump and adjusted to a value of about 50% of portal venous flow.

Removal of the Liver The preservation of the normal attachments of the perfused liver within the carcass facilitates free drainage of venous return owing to the support conferred by the attachment of the diaphragm to the inferior vena cava.

There are experiments where it is obligatory to remove the liver; for example, when it is required to measure continuously liver weight changes or obtain biopsies during perfusion.

Removal of the liver, where it may be necessary for the experiment, requires very careful attention to the suprahepatic inferior vena cava cannula, to avoid twisting, kinking or a flutter effect. The careful control of hepatic venous pressure to lie just below the hydrostatic pressure at the hilum seems to improve the alternate collapse and distension of the vena cava observed at lower hepatic venous pressures. Even short periods of impaired venous drainage may vitiate the preparation.

The surgical preparation before the start of perfusion is identical to that already described save for passing a thread ligature around the infrahepatic inferior vena cava. This enables easy ligation of the vessel at a later stage. In order to place the ligature between the lowest hepatic vein and the adrenal vein it is necessary to mobilise the right kidney – with the kidney dissected free from the posterior abdominal wall, a curved clamp can be passed behind the vena cava precisely under direct vision. When perfused via the portal vein and hepatic artery, the perfusate draining from both supra- and infra-hepatic inferior vena cava and isolated from all other organs, the liver can conveniently be excised.

This involves the division of the attachment of the diaphragm to the chest wall and vertebral column, leaving the liver held only by the supra- and infra-hepatic vena cava. Once the infra-hepatic vena cava has been ligated and divided, the liver can be removed to a special container.

Artery forceps are applied to the cut edges of the left cupola of the diaphragm and its attachment to the chest wall progressively divided in a posterior direction. The left cupola of the diaphragm is held to the right with forceps, allowing good exposure of the left crus and connective tissue attachments between aorta and diaphragm, which are then divided. Further retraction to the right reveals the right crus which is also cut across. The right cupola of the diaphragm is divided from the chest wall in a similar manner, thus completely freeing the diaphragm, with the liver attached, from the carcass. At this stage the liver is held vertically out of the wound by means of the forceps applied to the diaphragm, displaying the infrahepatic inferior vena cava with the surrounding ligature placed at an earlier stage in the procedure. This is tied, the infrahepatic venous drainage line simultaneously clamped and the vena cava divided below the level of the ligature. The liver can now be removed from the dog.

A suitable container is shown in Figure 12. Made of Perspex, the box can conveniently rest on a stand or spring balance, should continuous monitoring of weight changes be needed. Slots cut in the side allow the cannulae to and from the liver to lie securely. The preparation itself rests on a polythene sheet which is fixed transversely across the box. Perforations in the sheet permit the free drainage of clear fluid appearing on the liver surface. Cannulae inserted into the common bile duct or a lymphatic can be led through a slot and the secretion collected at a standard height with respect to the preparation. During an experiment where weight changes are being measured, the cannulae must be firmly supported, for example by clamps.

The whole container may be covered by a lid or polythene sheet, minimising evaporation and preventing desiccation of the liver surface.

Use has been made (Abouna, 1969) of a container equipped with a transverse artificial diaphragm which can be made to oscillate by alternate changes of externally applied pressure beneath it. The liver is placed on this diaphragm and it is suggested that the oscillation, simulating *in vivo* diaphragmatic movement during respiration, aids venous drainage. The use of a fibre-glass container moulded to the shape of the pig liver has been reported to improve venous drainage (Hobbs *et al,* 1968).

It has been found by trial and error that venous drainage is improved, with an associated fall in portal venous pressure, when the liver is placed with its diaphragmatic and anterior surfaces in contact with the polythene sheet and its visceral surface directed upwards.

Cannulation of Lymphatics Some of the studies which may be performed using the isolated canine liver require the creation of a lymph fistula.

Fig. 12

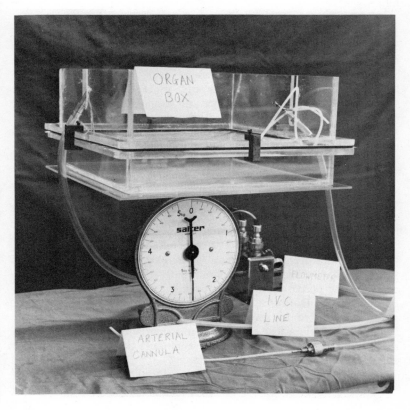

In the dog hepatic lymphatics leave the liver parenchyma at two different sites (Ritchie, 1956). Hilar lymphatics carrying about 80% of total hepatic lymph flow emerge alongside the portal veins embedded in the adventitia. Lymphatics draining the remaining 20% accompany the hepatic veins and pierce the diaphragm. Both systems drain into the main hepatic lymphatic cisterna chyli or thoracic duct. The hilar lymphatics may readily be cannulated. Before doing so the main hepatic lymphatic, receiving as tributaries all the hilar lymphatics, should be ligated, thus producing lymphatic engorgement. A large engorged lymphatic is selected, the adventitia cleaned from its surface over a distance of 0·5 to 1·0 cm and fine threads passed behind it. A longitudinal incision is made using fine ophthalmic scissors and a narrow-bore (1 mm internal diameter) firm polythene cannula inserted and tied in place. Lymph drains freely and can be collected at a standard level with respect to the hilum.

Monitoring
The continuous recording of certain parameters allows a simple, ready and immediate assessment of the preparation to be made.

Those parameters routinely measured include perfusing pressures, liver weight, bile flow, perfusate pH, pCO_2, PCV, porto/hepatic venous oxygen saturation difference and temperature.

To be suitable for physiological studies the preparation should be stable. During the first 60 minutes of perfusion certain changes in these parameters occur. By the end of this period values have become steady and usually remain so for the next 2–3 hours.

Portal venous, hepatic arterial and hepatic venous pressures are continuously measured, using manometry or by strain gauge transducers linked to a Mingograf 81 recorder.

The portal pressure is a most useful guide of a stable preparation free from outflow block. A steady pressure indicates an unchanging vascular resistance where flow is constant. Initially high, the portal pressure settles over 30–60 minutes to a value usually less than 10 cm water. Pressures above 15 cm continuing steadily to rise indicate a deteriorating preparation. This is usually the first sign of impending outflow block. During a satisfactory perfusion, portal pressure remains below 15 cm for several hours.

Lateral hepatic artery pressure is measured either at a point along the hepatic arterial cannula or from a cannula tied into the proximal end of the divided gastro-duodenal artery.

In perfused canine livers, the hepatic arterial pressure is lower than in the intact animal (180 mm Hg). This does not reflect inadequate flow rate, but is due to the reduced viscosity of the perfusate following dilution of the donor blood and probably sympathetic denervation and low levels of sympathomimetic hormones following exclusion of the adrenals. Values of around 100 mm Hg are usually obtained but this is variable. The hepatic artery pressure remains steady during perfusion even when portal venous flow is changed. The converse does not appear to apply; changes in arterial flow produce small but definite changes in portal venous pressures.

In the intact animal hepatic venous pressure lies just below atmospheric pressure (Greenaway and Stark, 1971). Brauer *et al* (1959) in their classic paper showed that congestive changes in the isolated perfused rat liver did not begin to occur until hepatic venous pressure was raised beyond hilar pressure. Even pressures as small as +1 cm of water caused rises in portal pressure, liver weight and tissue compartment size. The canine liver appears to be similar.

The hepatic venous pressure in the perfused canine liver can be changed passively by altering the height of the preparation relative to the level of the oxygenator. It is routinely adjusted to 4–5 cm water negative to the hilum and monitored using a saline manometer inserted into the side-arm of the venous outflow end-piece.

During any canine liver perfusion, the liver weight increases. In the first 2 hours this rise is small, usually at a rate of 10–20 g/hr. Once the portal pressure starts to rise, indicating an increasing hepatic resistance, then the rise in liver weight accelerates. By the end of 4 hours the liver weight may have risen by 20–30%, a figure of the same order as reported in the pig (Jablonski *et al*, 1971).

During the course of perfusion the haematocrit remains steady or increases slightly. It is adjusted by the addition of Krebs solution to 35 and monitored in each experiment.

In the perfusion system used, both the portal vein and hepatic arterial blood is fully oxygenated. The pO_2 is of the order of 200–400 mm Hg, corresponding to 100% haemoglobin saturation. At an adequate perfusion flow rate, the hepatic venous blood is usually about 60–70% saturated. Routine inflow and hepatic venous oxygen saturation estimations are made during each perfusion.

Temperature is monitored by a thermocouple, and is maintained at 38°C by means already described.

The pH and pCO_2 are monitored. At the start of perfusion, the portal venous pH is usually low with a standard bicarbonate of 15–22 mEq/L. Measurement of pH and pCO_2 is performed routinely at the beginning and the amount of added bicarbonate required is determined from the base deficit circulated from the Siggaard–Andersen nomogram and the volume of the perfusing medium.

Usually 10–30 mEq bicarbonate are needed initially while, during the first 120 minutes, 10 mEq may be required in addition.

Hepatic venous pH determinations range between 0·03 and 0·10 pH units below portal venous values.

Figure 13 shows monitoring parameters in a typical perfusion. Arterial or portal vein pH values ranging from 7·30 to 7·45 are compatible with a satisfactory preparation.

Perfusion flow rate is continuously monitored. The organ is perfused in a portal venous/hepatic artery ratio of 2:1. Total hepatic blood flow is adjusted to produce a hepatic venous O_2 saturation of 60–70%, this criterion is taken to indicate satisfactory perfusion (Ritchie et al, 1962).

In the canine liver, perfusion flow rates of 0·5–1·0 ml/g tissue/min have been used depending on the haematocrit. These flows are comparable to those used by other workers.

Hepatic Venous Outflow Block In the dog, especially, the condition known as hepatic venous outflow block presents a problem in liver perfusion.

At a variable time after the start of perfusion, the liver becomes gradually swollen, congested, cyanosed and blotchy. Clear fluid streams from the surface, portal pressure rises and bile flow diminishes. These changes are accompanied by a rise in liver weight and lymph flow, an increase of the red cell mass and expansion of the extracellular fluid space.

Once spontaneously engendered, this syndrome is irreversible, rendering the preparation useless for further studies.

Whereas Bauer et al (1932) found venous outflow block occurring within 30 minutes in their canine perfusions, advances over the subsequent 40 years have led to improved survival. It is now possible to perfuse the canine liver for several hours before serious deterioration occurs.

The changes characterising the syndrome of outflow block can all be reproduced by histamine. Its effect may, however, be reversible, resolving after 5–10 minutes with injected histamine in a dose of 20 μg.

Anaphylactoid shock or the intraparenchymal injection of extracts of ascaris suum cause identical changes in whole dogs (Thomas and Essex, 1949). A wide range of endotoxins and pharmacological agents have qualitatively similar effects (Greenaway and Stark, 1971).

A rise in hepatic venous pressure above the hydrostatic pressure of the hilum leads to the same changes. Provided passive venous congestion lasts no longer than about 10 minutes, the liver usually

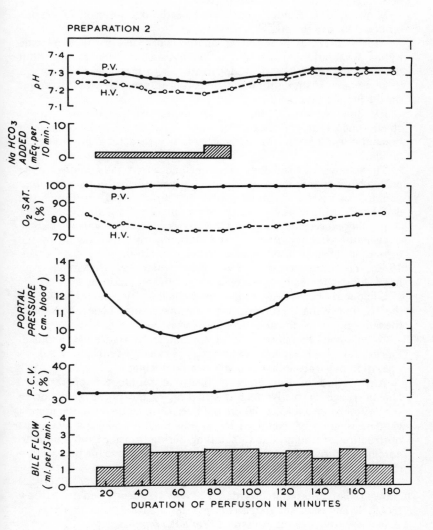

PREPARATION 2

Fig. 13 Methods of monitoring the preparation.

recovers but with periods extending much longer, the changes become permanent and deterioration progressive.

Many various factors seem to induce the development of venous outflow block in the dog.

Arey (1941) has provided an anatomical basis for this syndrome by his observations that in dog, seal and raccoon, there exists within the walls of small hepatic venous radicles to large hepatic veins, a large amount of smooth muscle. Spasm of this muscle would account for the picture described.

Extended survival of the perfused canine liver in recent years is chiefly due to the prevention of outflow block by adoption of certain precautions and the maintenance of a satisfactory physiological milieu.

The removal of vasoconstrictor substances from the non-disposable parts of the apparatus by the method already described is a *sine qua non* for successful perfusion. Adherent protein and other material deposited during a previous experiment must be eliminated.

In our experience early outflow block occurred when a bubble oxygenator (Pulmopak) was used. Possibly this was owing to the formation of denatured plasma protein microthrombi (Lee *et al*, 1961). The introduction of a roller oxygenator as used in the Aga heart–lung machine has greatly improved the preparations.

Silicone rubber is now used in preference to PVC tubing, owing to the possibility that vasoconstrictor substances may be leached out of the latter by the perfusate (Duke and Vane, 1968).

At all times handling of the liver should be rigorously avoided. During surgery, the liver may be gently packed away from the field of operation by swabs moistened with warmed Ringer.

Any period of ischaemia is likely to vitiate the preparation. Haemorrhage or inadvertent obstruction of the portal vein during surgery must be avoided. Where the liver is to be removed, the utmost gentleness must be exercised to prevent mechanical hepatic venous obstruction or trauma due to handling during transfer from animal to container. Early denervation of the liver may improve the preparation (Shoemaker *et al*, 1960).

It is essential to use autologous blood. Andrews *et al* (1955) showed that cross-matched donor blood frequently led to outflow block. It has been suggested (Eiseman *et al*, 1963) that this may be due to sensitivity to the parasite, *Dirofilaria immitis*.

Adequate anticoagulation must be ensured. A dose of 3 mg heparin/kg is given just before the start of perfusion, half intravenously and half into the reservoir. In our experience this dose of heparin appears to be inadequate after 3 hours. At this time, the addition of further heparin may reduce portal venous pressure. (Hardcastle, 1965).

Careful regulation of the pH is an important factor. Where the pH falls much below 7·30 evidence of increasing hepatic vascular resistance may be apparent. This should reverse on correcting pH to values between 7·30 and 7·45. By monitoring pH and pCO_2 during perfusion base deficit can be corrected by the addition of bicarbonate.

By reducing the haematocrit in the intact greyhound from its value of 60–70 to perfusate values of 30–40, it is our experience that flow characteristics are improved and red cell trauma lessened, with associated prolonged survival of the preparation.

Precautions to ensure adequate perfusion during the time of surgery have already been mentioned. The dog liver is particularly sensitive to periods of ischaemia. Once perfusion has been started portal flow should be increased to a satisfactory value within 15 minutes and the hepatic artery should be cannulated and perfused early.

Assessment

Many different tests are available for the assessment of function of the perfused liver. Most workers have used measurements of O_2 utilisation, bile flow, and clearance studies as satisfactory criteria of function. In addition biochemical tests may be performed directly on the bile and plasma and samples of tissue are available for histology or analysis of radio-isotopes in the measurement of tissue compartment size.

Oxygen Utilisation
There have been few reports of direct measurement of hepatic O_2 utilisation in intact animals. In dog under pentobarbital anaesthesia, a value of 5·66 ml/100 g liver/min has been reported (Selkurt and Brecher, 1956). Hepatic O_2 utilisation in man of 3·5 ml/100 g liver/min has been estimated from indirect measurements (Brauer, 1963).

In the isolated perfused liver O_2 utilisation is easily measured and similar values have been obtained by various workers using dog (Kestens *et al*, 1961; Hardcastle and Ritchie, 1968), pig (Eiseman *et al*, 1964; Hickman *et al*, 1971) and calf (Chapman *et al*, 1961). These range from 2–7 ml/100 g liver/min. A utilisation below 1 probably indicates a defective preparation. In the dog, values between 2·5–5·0 ml/100 g liver/min are usually expected.

Provided perfusion flow rate and the haemoglobin concentration are known the O_2 utilisation can be calculated knowing the O_2 saturation difference across the liver and where 1 gram of haemoglobin is equivalent to $1 \cdot 34$ ml O_2.

Towards the end of perfusion, the liver takes up less O_2, shown by an increasing hepatic venous saturation.

Before this terminal rise, the oxygen uptake by the liver usually remains steady in each experiment for several hours. This may be despite the presence of venous outflow block.

Hypothermia and metabolic inhibitors can be shown to arrest O_2 uptake whilst an ammonia load produces a rapid immediate increase of 10–20% (Hardcastle, 1965).

Bile

In the isolated perfused liver under basal conditions, bile is secreted at a steady rate. After the initial hour, during which the preparation becomes stable, bile flow remains steady for the next 2–4 hours. In the dog, bile flows at a rate of 8–12 ml/hr and under basal conditions consecutive collections at 15-minute intervals show little variation in volume.

At this flow rate, sufficient bile is available to make possible the determination of the concentration of bile constituents, e.g. bilirubin, bile salts, alkaline phosphatase, pH and electrolytes, and over a similar time course levels are steady. It is during this period that studies can be performed.

In the intact animal difficulties in cannulation of the common bile duct and the variation of exogenous influences, hormonal, nervous, and haemodynamic, may influence the bile and complicate the interpretation of results. The isolated perfused preparation is suitable for the investigation of bile flow and composition; there is greater exogenous control and mechanical obstruction to bile flow can be more easily remedied. In the next section data are presented to show how the preparation can be used for such a study.

Clearance Studies

Various substances introduced into the blood may be conjugated in the liver and excreted into the bile in a concentration several hundred times plasma levels. In the isolated perfused liver bromosulphalein (BSP) (Hardcastle and Ritchie, 1968; Chapman et al, 1961), indocyanine green (Hobbs et al, 1968) and rose bengal (Van Wyk et al, 1965) have been used to assess the function of the perfused liver.

In Figure 14 the clearance of BSP following a single loading dose of 150 mg is shown. Plasma values rapidly fall to levels of 1 mg %

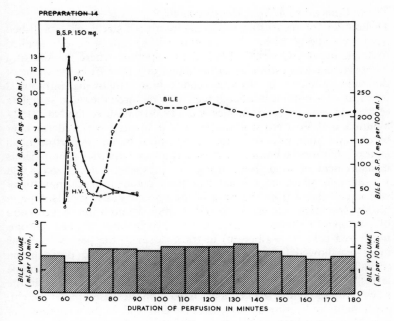

Fig. 14 B.S.P. clearance from the plasma and excretion in the bile.

whilst bile concentrations rise to a plateau of about 200 mg % after 30 minutes.

A steady continuous infusion of BSP at a rate of 1 mg per minute allows the same assessment of liver function, but avoids the sudden effect on bile flow that a single large dose is likely to produce.

The perfused liver rapidly clears an ammonia load entering the liver. During a 10-minute infusion of ammonia acetate at a rate of 12 mg/min into the portal vein, portal venous ammonia concentrations of 16–20 μg/ml were produced. Simultaneous measurement of levels in hepatic venous blood showed values never exceeding 3 μg/ml (Figure 15).

The infusion produces an immediate increase in O_2 utilisation by the liver of the order of 10–20%.

Measurement of the perfusate lactate/pyruvate ratio is a good indication of whether aerobic respiration is proceeding. In the isolated perfused canine liver, a steady ratio of 10–15 is usually found.

The clearance of a single loading dose of lactate fails to distinguish between anaerobic and aerobic respiration rate and is therefore less useful as a means of assessment.

Tissue Compartment Size Measurements

Techniques for measuring tissue compartment size, well established from whole-body studies (Moore *et al*, 1968), can be readily applied to single organs. Goresky (1963) used a method where the size of a compartment was estimated in the intact dog liver from the shape of the activity curve in hepatic venous blood following intraportal injection of a suitable labelled tracer. This required the rapid sampling of hepatic venous blood. Brauer *et al* (1959) measured the Na^{24}, I^{131}– albumin and Fe^{56} red cell spaces in the isolated perfused rat liver before and after passive venous congestion. In this department, an isotope dilution technique has been employed for the simultaneous measurement of total tissue water, inulin space, red cell mass and I^{131}–albumin space in the isolated perfused canine liver. Compartment size is calculated from the ratio of the specific activity of isotope in biopsy specimens compared to blood, after the addition of a mixture of isotopes (tritiated water, C^{14}-hydroxymethyl inulin, chromium^{51}–red cells, I^{131}–albumin) in trace doses to the perfusate. Time must be allowed for equilibration between blood and parenchyma (usually complete by 60 minutes as judged by hepatic lymph isotope levels). During the course of perfusion, there is a gradual rise in the sizes of these compartments, associated with increase in liver weight, presumably indicating a progressive oedema and, in the later stages of perfusion, red cell congestion.

Between 60–120 minutes, mean values of 78% for total tissue water and 25% for inulin space are seen. The preparation is suitable for the study of the effect of various stimuli e.g. haemodynamic changes of flow or pressure, differences in perfusate composition, biliary obstruction, pharmacological agents and metabolic inhibitors etc., on the size of tissue compartments.

Lymph Flow

The association between increased lymph flow and hepatic venous congestion is well known (Nix *et al*, 1951). It has proved possible to cannulate hilar lymphatics in the preparation, and data on lymph flow in the isolated perfused canine liver is available. A perfusion apparently satisfactory in all recorded parameters produces a steady flow of lymph comparable to flow and composition of hepatic lymph found in intact dogs (Cain *et al*, 1947). Increase of perfusing pressures and particularly hepatic venous pressure produces increased lymph flow. It would seem that a steady lymph flow is a sensitive indication that the haemodynamic status of the preparation is satisfactory. A rise in lymph flow may be the earliest indication of impending venous outflow block. It may also of course be affected in other ways (Figure

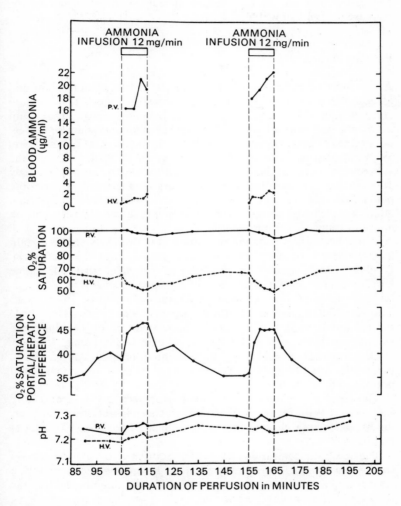

Fig. 15 Effect of ammonia acetate on the oxygen uptake of the isolated perfused canine liver.

16). The effect of doubling the portal venous flow on lymph flow and other parameters is shown. The change in weight suggests hepatic congestion and this in turn would appear to be the cause of the increase in lymph flow.

Plasma Constituents

At the start of perfusion, there is a resultant loss of potassium and glucose from the liver. This is shown above in Figure 2. Potassium concentrations in hepatic venous blood, having attained a maximum at 10 minutes, gradually fall as the liver takes up potassium so that by 60 minutes of perfusion steady levels usually below 4 mEq/L are seen. With glucose, maximum concentrations occur at 30 minutes and the subsequent uptake of glucose by the liver has usually been effected by 100 minutes. During the next 3–4 hours of a control preparation, potassium remains steady at 3–6 mEq/L while beyond 3 hours, addition of glucose to the perfusate may be required to keep plasma concentrations within normal limits.

It has been known for many years that a liver exposed to certain adverse stimuli releases potassium and glucose into the circulation. D'Silva (1936) showed in the isolated cat liver that adrenaline infusion caused an immediate liberation of potassium.

These findings are consistent with results obtained from intact animals (McChesney et al, 1949; Bearn et al, 1951; Ellis, 1951; Bloom and Russell, 1955) and can be reproduced by hepatic nerve stimulation (Hardcastle and Ritchie, 1968; Craig and Honig, 1963).

Haemorrhagic shock in the intact animal (Shoemaker et al, 1961), ischaemia and hypoxia cause a similar release of glucose and potassium from the liver.

The reverse phenomenon occurs during recovery following any such insult. With revascularisation after transplantation of the liver, the hypokalaemia induced may have clinical importance (Abouna et al, 1971).

The ionic concentrations of plasma sodium and chloride remain steady during the course of perfusion. Bicarbonate concentration which would otherwise fall can be artificially maintained by the addition of exogenous bicarbonate.

The preparation manufactures urea and this is seen by the increase in perfusate urea concentration. Figure 17 shows the mean rise in 5 separate liver perfusions over a period of 2 hours. Bilirubin and alkaline phosphatase levels remain within normal limits. Where biliary obstruction has been intentionally induced 30 minutes before

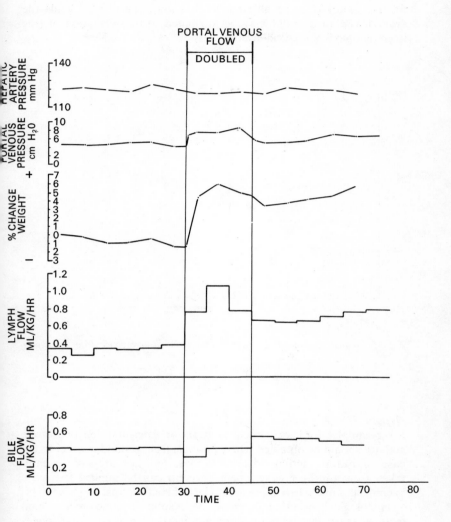

Fig. 16 The effect of doubling portal flow from 340 to 680 ml/min on hepatic artery and portal venous pressure, weight, lymph and bile flows, in the isolated perfused canine liver.

perfusion a rise in bilirubin and alkaline phosphatase is not detectable for 2–3 hours. Plasma albumin levels show little change while the gradual rise in globulin may be attributed to the formation of free haemoglobin from red cell trauma.

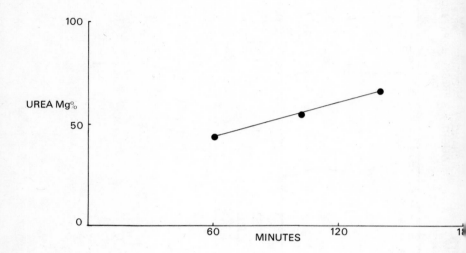

Fig. 17 Isolated perfused canine liver. Perfusing blood urea concentration 5 experiments.

Hepatic Tissue

Liver samples for biochemical analysis or determination of isotope activity should be obtained where possible from a standard site. In the case of isotope activity determinations, biopsies are conveniently taken from the liver edge where a clamp can be applied to secure haemostasis and where there are no large hepatic veins.

Histological examination may be helpful in assessment, such features as hepatocyte vacuolation and increase in intercellular spaces suggesting a degree of deterioration. Sections stained for glycogen may provide a qualitative means of estimating hepatocyte function, at least with respect to glycogen synthesis.

In Figures 18 and 19 are shown photomicrographs of low and high power sections of the same liver before and after 2 hours of perfusion.

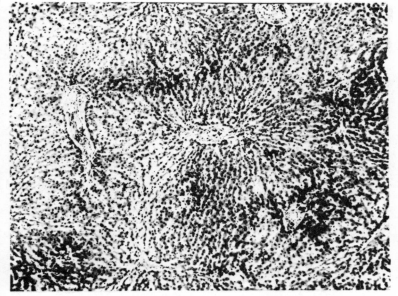

Fig. 18 Low power view of histological section of perfused liver.

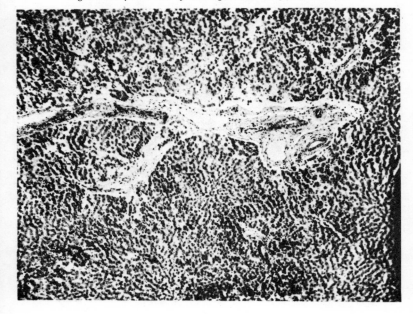

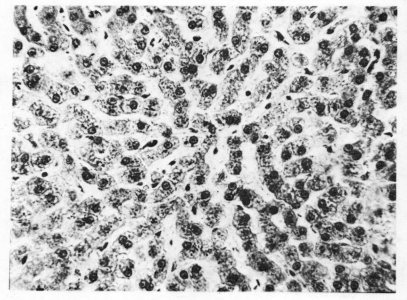

Fig. 19 High power view.

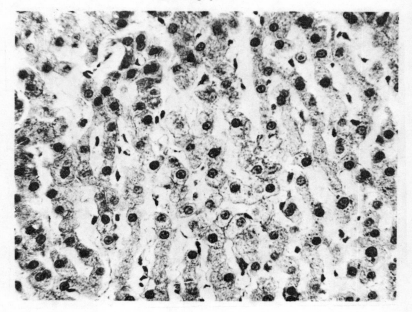

References

Abouna, G.M., Ashcroft, T., Hull, C., Hodson, A., Kirkley, J. and Walder, D.N. (1969) The assessment of function of the isolated perfused porcine liver. *Brit. J. Surg.* **56,** 289.

Abouna, G.M., Serrou, B., Boehning, H.G., Amemiya, H. and Martineau, G. (1970) Long-term support by intermittent multispecies liver perfusions. *Lancet* **ii,** 391.

Abouna, G.M., Aldrete, J.A. and Starzl, T.E. (1971) Changes in serum potassium and pH during clinical and experimental liver transplantation. *Surgery* **69,** 419.

Andrews, W.H.H. (1953) A technique for perfusion of the canine liver. *Ann. Trop. Med.* **47,** 146.

Andrews, W.H., Hecker, R., Maegraith, B.G. and Ritchie, H.D. (1955) The action of adrenaline, L-noradrenaline, acetylcholine and other substances on the blood vessels of the perfused canine liver. *J. Physiol.* **128,** 413.

Arey, L.B. (1941) Throttling veins in the livers of certain mammals. *Anat. Record.* **81,** 21.

Baer, R. and Roessler, R. (1926) Beiträge zur Pharmakologie der Lebergefässe *Arch. Exper. Path u. Pharmakol.* **119,** 204.

Bauer, W., Dale, H.H., Poulsson, L.T. and Richards, D.W. (1932) The control of circulation through the liver. *J. Physiol.* **74,** 343.

Bearn, A.G., Billing, B. and Sherlock, S. (1951) The effect of adrenaline and noradrenaline on hepatic blood flow and carbohydrate metabolism in man. *J. Physiol.* **115,** 430.

Bloom, W.L. and Russell, J.A. (1955) Effect of epinephrine and of norepinephrine on carbohydrate metabolism in the rat. *Am. J. Physiol.* **183,** 356.

Brauer, R.W., Pessotti, R.L. and Pizzolato, P. (1951) Isolated rat liver preparation. Bile production and other basic studies. *Proc. Soc. Exp. Biol. Med.* **78,** 174.

Brauer, R.W., Holloway, R.J. and Leong, G.F. (1959) Changes in liver function and structure due to experimental passive congestion under controlled hepatic vein pressures. *Amer. J. Physiol.* **197,** 681.

Brauer, R.W. (1963) Liver circulation and function. *Physiol. Rev.* **43,** 115.

Cain, J.C. *et al* (1947) Lymph from liver and thoracic duct. *Surgery Gynec. Obstet.* **85,** 559.

Chakravarti, M. and Tripod, J. (1940) The action in the perfused liver of acetylcholine, sympathomimetic substances and local anaesthetics. *J. Physiol.* **97,** 316.

Chapman, N.D., Goldsworthy, P.D., Vorwiler, W., Nyhus, L.M. and Martinis, A.J. (1961) The isolated perfused bovine liver. *J. Exp. Med.* **113,** 981.

Condon, R.E., Chapman, N.D., Nyhus, L.M. and Harkins, H.N. (1960) Hepatic arterial and portal venous pressure-flow relationships in the isolated perfused liver. *Am. J. Physiol.* **202,** 1090.

Craig, A.B. and Honig, R.C. (1963) Hepatic metabolic and vascular responses to epinephrine: a unifying hypothesis. *Am. J. Physiol.* **205,** 1132.

Dale, H.H. (1929) Croonian lectures on some chemical factors in the control of circulation. *Lancet* **i,** 1180.

D'Silva, J.L. (1936) Action of adrenaline and serum potassium. *J. Physiol.* **86,** 219.

Duke, H.N. and Vane, J.R. (1968) An adverse effect of PVC tubing used in extracorporeal circulation. *Lancet* **ii,** 21.

Eiseman, B., Knipe, P., Koh, Y., Normell, L. and Spencer, F.C. (1963) Factors affecting hepatic vascular resistance in the perfused liver. *Ann. Surg.* **157,** 532.

Eiseman, B., Moore, T.C. and Normell, L. (1964) Histamine metabolism in the isolated perfused pig liver. *Surgery Gynec. Obstet.* **118,** 69.

Eiseman, B., Leim, D.S. and Raffucci, F. (1965) Heterologous liver perfusion in treatment of hepatic failure. *Ann. Surg.* **162,** 329.

Ellis, S. (1951) The effect of amines on the blood sugar of the rat. *J. Pharmac. Exp. Ther.* **101,** 92.

Goresky, C.A. (1963) A linear method for determining sinusoidal and extravascular volumes. *Am. J. Physiol.* **204,** 626.

Greenaway, C.V. and Stark, R.D. (1971) The hepatic vascular bed. *Physiol. Rev.* **51,** 23.

Hardcastle, J.D. (1965) Glucose and potassium exchange between the isolated canine liver and perfusing blood. M.Chir. Thesis. Cantab.

Hardcastle, J.D. and Ritchie, H.D. (1967) The liver in shock (1). *Brit. J. Surg.* **54,** 679.

Hardcastle, J.D. and Ritchie, H.D. (1968) The liver in shock (2). *Brit. J. Surg.* **55,** 365.

Hickman, R., Saunders, S.J., Simson, E. and Terblanche, J. (1971) Perfusion of the pig liver. *Brit. J. Surg.* **58,** 33.

Hobbs, K.E.F., Hunt, A.C., Palmer, D.B., Badrick, F.E., Morris, A.M., Mitra, S.K., Peacock, J.H., Immelman, E.J. and Riddell, A.G. (1968) Hypothermic low flow liver perfusion as a means of porcine hepatic storage for 6 hours. *Brit. J. Surg.* **55,** 696.

Jablonski, P., Douglas, M.C., Gordon, E., Owen, J.A. and Watts, J.McK. (1971) Studies on the isolated perfused pig liver. *Brit. J. Surg.* **58,** 129.

Kestens, P.J., Farrelly, J.A. and McDermott, W.V. (1961) A technique of isolation and perfusion of the canine liver. *J. Surg. Res.* **1,** 58.

Lee, W.H., Krumhaar, D., Fonkalsrud, E.W., Schjeide, O.A. and Maloney, J.V. (1961) Denaturation of plasma proteins as a cause of morbidity and death after intracardiac operations. *Surgery* **50,** 29.

McChesney, E.W., McAuliffe, J.P. and Blumberg, H. (1949) The hyperglycaemic action of some analogs of epinephrine. *Proc. Soc. Exp. Biol. Med.* **71,** 220.

McLaughlin, A.R. (1928) The role of the liver in controlling the distribution of blood. *J. Pharmacol.* **34,** 147.

Mautner, H. and Pick, E.P. (1915) Uber die durch Schockgifte erzeugten Zirkulations storungen. *Munchner Medizin Wehnschrift Bd* **62,** S1141.

Moore, F.D., Hartsuck, J.M., Zollinger, R.M. Jr., and Johnson, J.E. (1968) Reference models for clinical studies by isotope dilution. *Ann. Surg.* **168,** 671.

Nix, J.T., Mann, F.C., Bollman, J.L., Grindlay, J.H. and Flock, E.V. (1951) Alteration of protein constituents of lymph by specific injury to liver. *Amer. J. Physiol.* **164,** 119.

Ritchie, H.D. (1956) Surgical jaundice: An experimental study. M.Ch. Thesis. Edinburgh.

Ritchie, H.D., Freeman, M.A.R. and Shaw, D. (1962) The value of rapid blood oxygen saturation determination during heart-lung bypass experiments. *J. Roy. Coll. Surg. Edin.* **7,** 295.

Selkurt, E.E. and Brecher, G.A. (1956) Splanchnic haemodynamics and oxygen utilisation during haemorrhagic shock in dog. *Circ. Res.* **4,** 693.

Shoemaker, W.C., Panico, F.G., Walker, W.F. and Elwyn, D.H. (1960) Perfusion of canine liver *in vivo*. *J. Appl. Physiol.* **15,** 687.

Shoemaker, W.C., Walker, W.F. and Turk, L.N. (1961) The role of the liver in the development of haemorrhagic shock. *Surgery Gynec. Obstet.* **112,** 327.

Simonds, J.P. and Brandes, W.W. (1929) The effect of peptone on the hepatic veins in the dog. *J. Pharmacol.* **35**, 165.

Thomas, W.D. and Essex, H.E. (1949) Observations on the hepatic venous circulation with special reference to sphincteric mechanism. *Amer. J. Physiol.* **158**, 303.

Trowell, O.A. (1942) Urea formation in the isolated perfused liver of the rat. *J. Physiol.* **100**, 432.

Van Wyk, J., Leim, D.S. and Eiseman, B. (1965) Function of cadaver liver. *Surgery* **58**, 120.

Anaesthesia and the Isolated Liver

Introduction

The isolated liver permits investigation of the effects of anaesthetic agents on the liver, metabolism of such drugs by the liver and the metabolic functions of the liver under normal and abnormal physiological conditions. These include changes in blood flow rate, oxygenation, acid-base balance and temperature. In addition, prior to perfusion the whole animal may be subjected to multiple anaesthetics (Biebuyck *et al,* 1970) or the liver microsomal enzymes responsible for drug metabolism may be induced or inhibited by drug therapy (Scholler, 1971). Liver damage or biliary obstruction may be produced by drugs or surgery and the isolated damaged liver studied during subsequent perfusion. For the anaesthetist therefore, this preparation offers an opportunity to investigate under controlled conditions a variety of problems pertinent to clinical practice.

In general terms, liver perfusion preparations can be divided into large – such as dog, pig, calf; and small – such as rat. The advantages and disadvantages of these are discussed in detail in the chapter – Choice of Animal. We have preferred a large liver (dog) because this permits a big volume of perfusate and therefore enables simultaneous withdrawal of multiple arterial and venous samples for evidence of uptake or release by the liver of electrolytes, enzymes, injected materials etc., without excessive dilution of the substances under study. Some work from our laboratory is now presented as an illustration of the range of studies which can be carried out with this preparation.

Volatile Agents

Direct Effects
Volatile anaesthetic agents may be introduced into the blood (perfusate) by passing the oxygenator gas through a calibrated vaporiser.
The actual blood concentration produced should be measured by gas
chromatography. It is then possible, for comparative studies, to adjust
the vaporiser to give blood levels comparable with those of the
anaesthetised intact animal. Before introducing inflammable or explosive agents into the oxygenator, care should be taken that the
perfusion system is spark-proof.

In addition to standard tests of liver function, the isolated liver has
the advantage that measurements which are not possible in the intact
animal, such as glucose and potassium balance studies, may be made.
Each perfusion acts as its own control as observations may be
performed before, during and after a period of exposure to a volatile
agent. For example, Figure 20 shows the effects of chloroform on
bromsulphthalein clearance; the depression of clearance is obvious
when compared with the control injection. Changes induced during
the period of anaesthesia may be followed into the recovery period.
Figure 21 shows the effects of chloroform on glucose and potassium
levels in the perfusate; note the loss of glucose from the liver occurring
during exposure to chloroform and the subsequent loss of potassium.

Enzyme levels are commonly used to assess liver function in the
intact animal. As there is no single enzyme which is specific to the
liver it is usual to study a wide range of cytoplasmic and mito-
chondrial enzymes in order to build up a pattern. Even so, changes
are difficult to interpret and may in fact reflect defects in organs other
than the liver. In the isolated liver however no other source is present
and study of the more easily measured enzymes such as aspartate
aminotransferase (GOT), is all that seems to be required for an
assessment of enzyme activity.

It is of interest that because the perfusion circuit is a closed system,
urea and aspartate aminotransferase show a steady rise with time in
the perfusate. No such rise is seen in alkaline phosphatase. During
administration of volatile anaesthetics there is inhibition of urea
production and often that of aspartate aminotransferase. Subsequently marked differences may be seen in the production of
aspartate aminotransferase (Figures 22, 23).

Any number of parameters may be observed and the effects of
volatile agents on these assessed. Table 2 shows the effects of
chloroform, methoxyflurane and halothane under conditions of
normal flow and oxygenation on a variety of measurements.

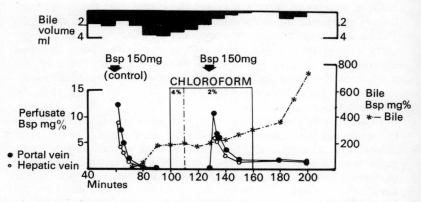

Fig. 20 Isolated canine liver: Effects of chloroform on bile secretion and brom-sulphthalein (Bsp) clearance from the perfusate and excretion in the bile.

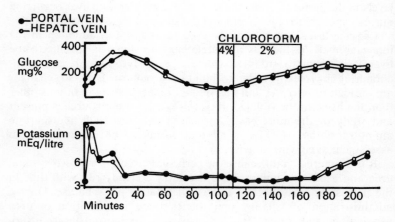

Fig. 21 Isolated canine liver: Effects of chloroform on glucose and potassium exchange between the perfusate and the liver.

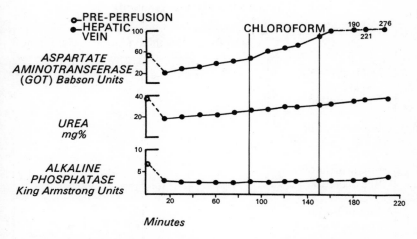

Fig. 22 *Isolated canine liver: Effects of chloroform on aspartate aminotransferase (GOT), urea and alkaline phosphatase in hepatic venous blood.*

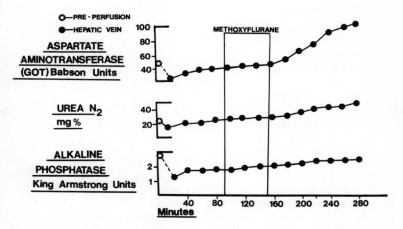

Fig. 23 *Isolated canine liver: Effects of methoxyflurane on aspartate aminotransferase (GOT), urea and alkaline phosphatase in hepatic venous blood.*

Table 2   Effects of Chloroform, Methoxyflurane and
Halothane on the Isolated Perfused Canine Liver
(Normal Flow and Oxygenation)

	Chloroform	Methoxyflurane	Halothane
Depression of Oxygen Consumption	+ +	+	+
Impairment of B.S.P. Clearance	+ +	+ +	+
Impairment of Bile Secretion	+ + +	+ +	–
Rise in Portal Venous Pressure	+ + +	+	–
Loss of Glucose from the Liver	+ + +	+ +	–
Loss of Potassium from the Liver	+ + +	+	–
Rise in Lactate/ Pyruvate Ratio	+ + +	+	–

Key {
   – No Effect
   + Slight Effect
  ++ Moderate Effect
+++ Severe Effect
}

Metabolism

Most volatile agents are metabolised in part by the liver and it has
been suggested that non-volatile metabolites may be hepatotoxic
(Cohen, 1971). As Klatskin (1969) has defined a hepatotoxic drug as
one capable of producing adverse changes in the experimental animal
as well as man, the isolated liver is an ideal preparation for the study
of such drugs.

Figure 24 shows the changes seen when $20\mu C$ ^{14}C halothane is
injected into the perfusate of a preparation after exposure to 2%

halothane for 30 minutes. It can be seen that non-volatile material appears in the perfusate within ten minutes and both volatile and non-volatile materials are excreted in the bile. The non-volatile material has been identified as trifluroacetic acid and trifluro-ethanolamide (Cohen, 1971).

The isolated preparation also allows study of the possible inhibition of metabolism of a drug by itself. Figure 24 showed the effects of ^{14}C halothane metabolism after a period of exposure of the preparation to high blood concentrations of halothane (approx. 40 mg/100 ml). Non-volatile material has nevertheless appeared after ten minutes,

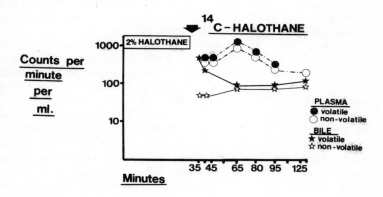

Fig. 24 Isolated canine liver: Metabolism of ^{14}C-halothane. Volatile and non-volatile material in plasma and bile.

indicating that under normal flow conditions in the isolated canine liver halothane metabolism occurs. This is in contrast to evidence from the intact pig (Sawyer *et al*, 1971) where halothane appears to inhibit its own metabolism. In the intact animal, however, liver blood flow can neither be controlled nor easily measured. It may be therefore that this metabolic inhibition is merely a reflection of reduced liver blood flow.

Biliary Obstruction and Anaesthetic Agents

In a series of dogs biliary obstruction was produced by ligation of the cystic and common bile ducts one week prior to liver perfusion. Severe changes in liver function tests were seen in control experiments (Table 3). During perfusion the biliary system was left obstructed.

Exposure to halothane at this stage did not produce further deterioration as measured by these and other tests.

Portal pressure was higher than in unobstructed perfusions and was more markedly affected by muscle relaxants. Figure 25 shows the effect of gallamine and halothane on portal pressure. A period of reduced liver blood flow was included in these studies to demonstrate that portal pressure could be reduced.

Muscle Relaxants

These drugs are commonly employed in anaesthesia. The isolated liver may be used to study two aspects; firstly histamine release and secondly metabolism and excretion in the bile.

The canine liver is very sensitive to histamine, although capable of metabolising it extremely efficiently. When histamine is injected into either the portal vein or hepatic artery there is a rise in portal pressure and an initial fall and subsequent rise in hepatic artery pressure (Figure 26). Figure 27 shows the effects of various muscle relaxants on portal and hepatic artery pressures. The transient effect of suxamethonium is due to its rapid metabolism by plasma cholinesterase. Pancuronium and alcuronium have a minimal effect on the hepatic vasculature (Figure 28). Some muscle relaxants do not release histamine but may have a cholinergic effect (Simpson *et al*, 1972). This is demonstrated by blockage of the vascular response by atropine but not by an antihistamine.

Metabolism of muscle relaxants, other than suxamethonium, is a slow process. Normally they are mainly excreted unchanged in the urine and to a small extent in the bile. In renal failure however, the choice of muscle relaxant may be influenced by knowledge of its metabolism and excretion.

^{14}C-pancuronium bromide and ^{14}C-tubocurarine were added to the perfusate of isolated canine liver perfusions (Figure 29). ^{14}C-pancuronium was cleared exponentially from the perfusate and appeared in the bile. Thin layer chromatography of the perfusate showed that there was probably a metabolite which appeared ten minutes after addition of the pancuronium. The perfusate level of ^{14}C-tubocurarine fell after ten minutes to a steady value which then remained stable for the rest of the period of study. Some tubocurarine was excreted into the bile but this was a slower process than with pancuronium. Although in the intact animal enterohepatic recirculation may reduce the effectiveness of biliary secretion as an excretion route; if however other routes of excretion fail, then the amount of a drug secreted in the bile may become clinically significant.

Table 3   Liver Function Tests One Week
after Biliary Obstruction in the Dog

	Alkaline Phosphatase (King Armstrong Units)	Bilirubin (mg %)	Aspartate Amino-transferase (Got – Babson Units)
1	465	52	990
2	484	33	287
3	466	40	480
4	267	36	274

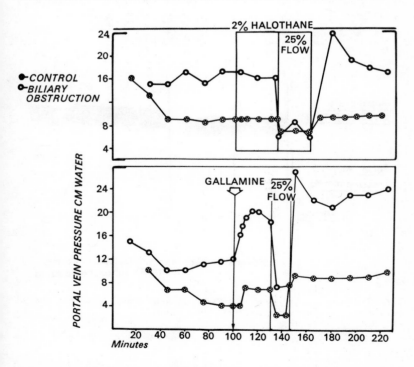

Fig. 25 Isolated canine liver: Effects of halothane, gallamine and reduced liver blood flow rate on portal vein pressure – control and biliary obstruction.

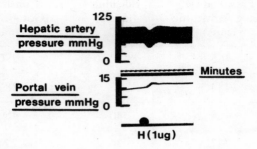

Fig. 26 Isolated canine liver: Effects of histamine (H) on hepatic artery and portal vein pressure.

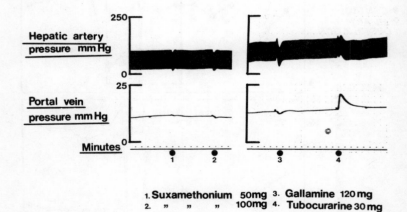

1. Suxamethonium 50mg 3. Gallamine 120 mg
2.   "   "   "   100mg 4. Tubocurarine 30 mg

Fig. 27 Isolated canine liver: Effects of suxamethonium, gallamine and d-tubocurarine on hepatic artery and portal vein pressure.

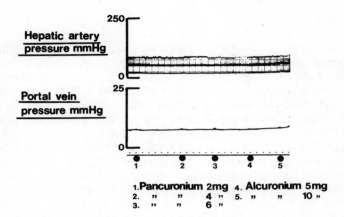

Fig. 28: Isolated canine liver: Effects of pancuronium and alcuronium on hepatic artery and portal vein pressure.

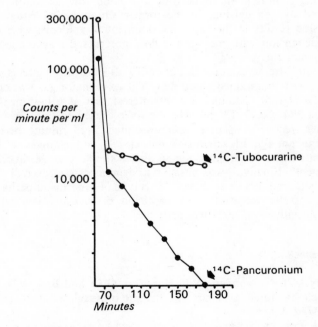

Fig. 29 Isolated canine liver: Clearance of ^{14}C-tubocurarine and ^{14}C-pancuronium from the perfusate.

Hypoxia

Hypoxia is one of the factors which may contribute to liver damage following anaesthesia. The isolated liver provides a model for the study of the effects of anaesthetic agents under conditions where the degree of hypoxia may be varied but other factors, such as blood flow rate and acid-base balance, are held constant.

A series of control experiments was carried out with a period of hypoxia induced either by reduced liver blood flow or reduced oxygen tension. This study confirmed the findings of Hardcastle and Ritchie (1967) who demonstrated loss of glucose and potassium from the liver. Subsequently comparable degrees of hypoxia were superimposed on livers exposed to halothane and methoxyflurane. The adverse biochemical effects were not greater than those seen in the control experiments. These findings suggest that when liver damage occurs in clinical practice in association with hypoxia and anaesthesia other factors must be involved.

A differentiation should be made between the degree of insult resulting from hypoxia induced by low blood flow, as compared with lowered oxygen tension. In the former situation, inadequate tissue perfusion results in the rapid development of acidosis, whereas low oxygen tension with maintained flow prevents the accumulation of local metabolites.

As an extreme example Iles *et al* (1972) studied the effects of total anoxia with maintained blood flow. The oxygenator gas was changed to 95% N_2:5% CO_2 and it is of interest that at a low measurable arterial PO_2 i.e. 7–13 mm Hg the liver ceased to take up oxygen. Further, recovery occurred after repeated 5–15 minute periods of absolute anoxia. Elevated succinate levels and changes in lactate pyruvate ratios occurred which paralleled similar changes in critically ill patients. Finally, it was possible to demonstrate a reversal of steps in the tricarboxycylic acid cycle. This type of experiment perhaps best illustrates the versatility and precision of measurement which is possible with an isolated liver perfusion.

References

Biebuyck, J.F., Saunders, S.J., Harrison, G.G. and Bull, A.B. (1970) Multiple halothane exposure and hepatic bromsulphthalein clearance. *Brit. Med. J.* **1,** 668.

Cohen, E.N. (1971) Metabolism of the volatile anesthetics. *Anesthesiology*, **35,** 193.

Hardcastle, J.D. and Ritchie, H.D. (1967) The liver in shock. *Brit. J. Surg.* **54,** 679.

Iles, R.A., Barnett, D., Strunin, L., Strunin, J.M., Simpson, B.R. and Cohen, R.D. (1972) The effect of hypoxia on succinate metabolism in man and the isolated perfused dog liver. *Clin. Sci.,* **42,** 35.

Klatskin, G. (1969) In *Diseases of the Liver.* ed. Schiff 3rd Ed. Philadelphia and Toronto, Lippincott.

Sawyer, D.C., Eger, E.I. II., Bahlman, S.H. (1971) Concentration dependence of hepatic halothane metabolism. *Anesthesiology,* **34,** 230.

Scholler, K.L. (1971) Modification of the effects of chloroform on the rat liver. *Brit. J. Anaesth.* **42,** 603.

Simpson, B.R., Strunin, L., Savege, T.M., Walton, B., Foley, E.I., Maxwell, M.P., Ross, L.A. and Harris, D.M. (1972) An azobisarylimidazo-pyridinium derivative: a rapidly acting non-depolarising muscle relaxant. *Lancet* **i,** 516.

The Isolated Perfused Porcine Liver

The technique used to perfuse the porcine liver is a modification of that employed for experiments with the canine liver. During the operation, anoxia to the liver is avoided in the same way as for the canine preparations. The blood volume of the pig used is smaller than that of the greyhound of similar weight, so that autologous sanguineous perfusion can only be successful if care is taken to prevent blood pooling in other abdominal organs such as the spleen and intestines. This can be achieved by ligating the splenic artery and superior mesenteric artery at appropriate moments in the course of the operation. The porcine liver preparation was used to study the effect of various substances on bile flow, and make comparison with effects observed with the same substances in the canine liver.

The Circuit

The circuit is similar to that used in the canine experiments. The main systemic blood vessels of the pig however are smaller than those of the dog and therefore require finer cannulae. The femoral vessels in articular are very small so that in the porcine experiments it is more satisfactory to insert a single venous cannula, to drain the hepatic veins directly into the inferior vena cava, and thereby dispense with dissection and cannulation of the femoral veins in the groins. Similarly a single cannula for bleeding the animal is inserted into the abdominal aorta in preference to the two cannulae normally placed in the femoral arteries of the dog.

The Anaesthetic

Pigs weighing between 17 and 27 kg are anaesthetised with halothane and oxygen by a mask applied to the snout. Sometimes it is necessary to pass an endotracheal tube in order to ensure that the airway is patent. The animal is allowed to breathe spontaneously during the operation. An inhalation anaesthetic agent is used in preference to thiopentone because venepuncture is particularly difficult in the pig.

The Operation

The pig is secured supine on the operating table. A midline incision is made from the xiphisternum to the pubis to allow sufficient exposure of the abdominal contents without any need to open the chest at this stage. The exposure is easier in the pig than the dog because the former tends to have a wider subcostal angle. The initial part of the operation is devoted to dissecting the relevant blood vessels and partially isolating the liver circulation without interfering with the portal venous and hepatic arterial flow into the liver. When this stage is complete the hepatic vessels themselves can be cannulated and perfused.

The abdominal aorta and inferior vena cava are sought above and below their bifurcations and cannulated. The aortic cannula is placed just inside the aorta and secured, and its distal end is led into the reservoir of the circuit; the venous cannula is passed up the inferior vena cava until its tip lies close to the entrance of the inferior hepatic veins. The aortic cannula will in due course provide the means for bleeding the pig to prime the perfusate with blood, and finally to exsanguinate the animal. The vena cava catheter will be used to drain blood from the liver in the early stages of perfusion.

An initial attempt to prevent loss of blood into the spleen and gastro-intestinal tract can be made by ligating the splenic artery and the left gastric artery. The former may be followed by splenectomy after the spleen has been seen to contract in size, but the latter vessel need only be ligated in continuity at this stage. It is often convenient at this point to transect the lower oesophagus between stout linen tapes. Large vessels in the gastro-hepatic omentum may also be ligated and transected, and one such vessel can be used to provide a channel for the measurement of hepatic arterial pressure when the perfusion has been set up. Care should be taken to avoid damaging the common bile duct, which is best left undisturbed until later.

The liver is now retracted under the protection of gauze swabs to avoid damage. The portal vein is usually more accessible in the pig than in the dog, so that it can itself be dissected from the lesser omentum and loosely surrounded by two thread ligatures as a preliminary to cannulation. The hepatic artery is sought as it emerges from the coeliac axis and is prepared in the same way.

Heparin (200 I.U. per kilogram body weight) is now injected into the animal and the circuit is primed with about 500 ml of blood released from the aortic cannula as in the case of the dog. The blood flow to the upper part of the gastro-intestinal tract is further reduced at this stage by applying a clamp across the superior mesenteric artery. When the portal cannula has been filled with blood-stained perfusate by temporarily turning on the appropriate pump, it can be inserted into the portal vein and secured by the previously applied ligatures. The portal vein pump can then be switched on and the inferior vena caval cannula clamp released so that the liver perfusion is commenced. The aortic cannula is also released to bleed the animal. During this time the hepatic artery has been perfused with the pig's own blood, but following the release of the inferior vena caval cannula and aortic clamp cardiac asystole usually occurs. Now the hepatic artery can be cannulated and perfused by the artificial circulation.

Next the thorax is opened by extending the initial abdominal incision to split the sternum. The other limb of the venous drainage cannula is inserted into the supradiaphragmatic part of the inferior vena cava and led out of the chest through an intercostal space. The liver is now being completely perfused by the artificial circuit. For the experiments performed using this preparation the liver remained *in situ* in the carcass and was not removed to be placed in a container. The preparation is finally established when the liver has been fully isolated from the gastro-intestinal tract and the biliary tree has been cannulated.

The common bile duct is identified, to be dissected and cannulated. This cannulation is performed at a late stage in the operation to minimise the chance of the cannula causing haemorrhage into the bile by abrading the mucosa of the duct. The cannula is led through the abdominal wall and its tip placed in a graduated tube placed at a lower level than the porta hepatis. The cystic duct is ligated or sutured, depending upon its accessibility; care being taken not to injure the liver at this point. The remaining vessels in the hepato-gastric and hepato-duodenal ligaments are ligatured and the intestinal tract removed from the carcass. The portal vein and hepatic artery pressure manometers are then set up.

The perfusate used in liver perfusion in the pig has a lower packed cell volume (P.C.V.) than that in the canine preparation. The initial P.C.V. of the pig's blood is approximately 40% and this is finally diluted by the Krebs solution in the circuit to 15% with a haemoglobin concentration of about 5 grams per 100 ml. The solution is too weak for its oxygen saturation to be determined by the methods used in the study of the canine liver, but experience has shown that the liver can be maintained in a satisfactory condition for experiments to be performed over a period of several hours. Hepatic venous outflow block does not appear to be a particular hazard in this species. For this reason and also because the tissues are easier to dissect, a satisfactory porcine liver perfusion can often be prepared more easily with the porcine liver than with that of the dog.

Studies of Bile Flow

The isolated porcine liver perfusion prepared by the method described has been shown to provide a satisfactory method for the study of the direct effect of various substances on bile flow. Bile appears to flow steadily at a rate of 15 ml per hour (0·65 ml per kg body weight per hour) so that bile is secreted in sufficient volume to allow several biochemical investigations to be made on specimens collected at frequent intervals. Since the methods used to perfuse the livers of the dog and pig are similar, experiments can be conducted to examine possible species differences in response to the same substance.

In our study of the effect of various substances on the flow and chemical composition of hepatic bile, several variables were measured. Such variables included the portal vein pressure and hepatic artery pressure of the liver; the volume of bile secreted every five minutes and its content of chloride, bicarbonate, bilirubin, cholate and alkaline phosphatase. Changes in bilirubin excretion can be reflected by infusing Bromosulphophthalein (B.S.P.) into the circuit and measuring the concentration of B.S.P. in the bile. These two substances are handled in much the same way by the liver (Lester and Troxler, 1969).

In Figure 30 observations from two porcine liver perfusions are superimposed. In each experiment Pentagastrin (200 microg), Sodium taurocholate (100 mg), Pentagastrin (300 microg) and Secretin (50 units) were administered in rotation and various observations were made. B.S.P. was infused into the perfusate at a rate of 1 mg per

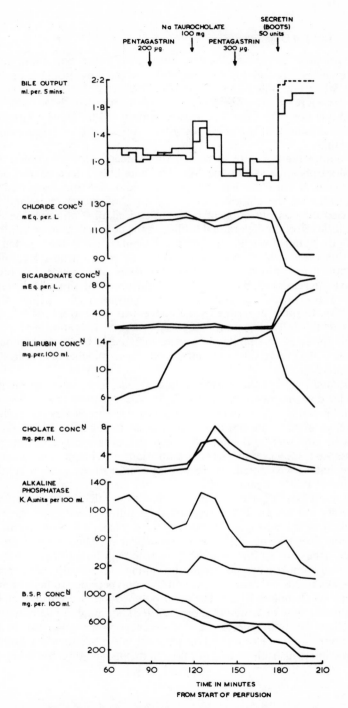

Fig. 30 The effect of pentagastrin, sodium taurocholate and secretin on bile flow and composition in two isolated perfused porcine liver preparations.

minute after an initial loading dose of 250 mg had been given. Pentagastrin appeared to have no effect on bile flow from the porcine liver when administered in these two different doses. Sodium taurocholate increased the bile flow, and the injections of Secretin stimulated bile flow when the liver had been perfused for three hours, thus demonstrating that the preparation was still capable of responding at this stage.

Sodium taurocholate increased the concentration of cholate and alkaline phosphatase in the bile, but had little effect on the other biochemical variables which were measured. Secretin decreased the concentration of chloride, increased that of bicarbonate and decreased the concentration of bilirubin and alkaline phosphatase, and had little effect on the gradual decline in the concentration of B.S.P.

In the canine liver, Pentagastrin in a similar dose to that used in the pig increased bile flow (Figure 31). There was a transitory fall in hepatic artery pressure. The concentrations of chloride and bicarbonate increased slightly and those of bilirubin and cholate fell. There was a transitory increase in the concentration of alkaline phosphatase. In other experiments the concentration of B.S.P. in bile was seen to fall following administration of B.S.P. Secretin, in the dose used, appeared to stimulate a greater increase in bile flow, and had a similar, but more marked, effect on these biochemical variables (Figure 32).

Sodium taurocholate also stimulated bile flow, when given in a similar dose, in the dog (Figure 33). It caused a transitory increase in portal pressure and a fall in hepatic artery pressure. There was a slight increase in the concentration of chloride to the bile, and a fall in bicarbonate; there was minimal change in bilirubin concentration, but a marked increase in the concentration of cholate and alkaline phosphatase was noted. There was also marked increase in concentration of B.S.P. (Beaugié, 1972).

It therefore appeared that bile flow from the isolated perfused porcine and canine livers responded in different ways to the substances tested when similar doses were used. Bile flow from the porcine liver was not affected by Pentagastrin when administered on seven occasions to four preparations in four different doses, whereas bile was stimulated to flow from the canine liver. Comparable results were obtained with another gastrin-like polypeptide studied, namely Caerulein (Beaugié, 1972). The other polypeptide, Secretin, which has a different type of structure (Jorpes, 1968), stimulated bile flow from the liver of both species, but differences were observed in the concentration of chloride and bicarbonate in the bile secreted. Sodium taurocholate also stimulated bile flow in the pig and dog, but in the pig

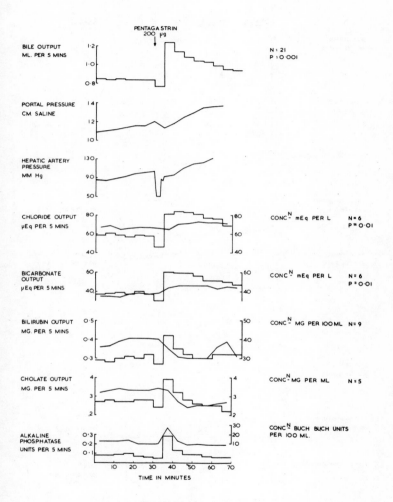

Fig. 31 *The effect of pentagastrin on bile flow and composition in the isolated perfused canine liver (Means from 21 experiments in 15 livers).*

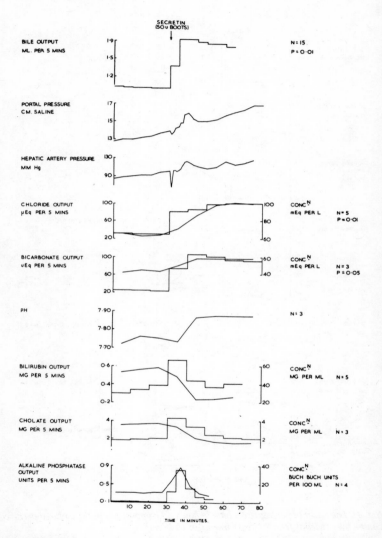

Fig. 32 The effect of secretin on bile flow and composition in the isolated perfused canine liver (Means from 15 experiments in 13 livers)

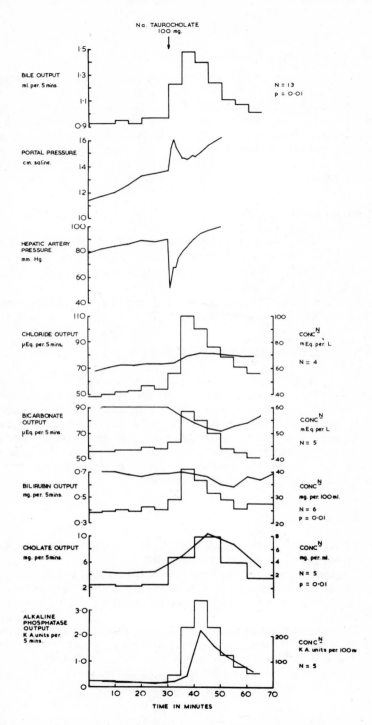

Fig. 33 The effect of sodium taurocholate on bile flow and composition in the isolated perfused canine liver (Means from 13 experiments in 13 livers).

had little effect on its chloride and bicarbonate content and no effect on B.S.P.

The isolated perfused porcine liver has therefore been a useful tool in a study of the effect of various substances on bile flow. It has enabled us to broaden our view of the effect of these substances by submitting them to another species and examining the different responses. Since the technique described is similar to that used in the dog, technical variables are unlikely to have influenced the results.

References

Lester, R. and Troxler, R.F. (1969) Recent advances in bile pigment metabolism. *Gastro-enterology* **56,** 143.

Beaugié, J.M. (1972) Gastro-duodenal hormones and bile flow. *Ann. Roy. Coll. Surg.* **50,** 164.

Jorpes, J.E. (1968) The isolation and chemistry of secretin and cholecystokin. *Gastro-enterology* **55,** 157.

Perfusion of the Isolated Rat Liver

Perfusion of the isolated rat liver was first reported by Corey and Britton (1941). During the last decade this preparation has become increasingly popular, especially in the investigation of metabolic pathways within the liver itself. It may be helpful to the reader to start by enumerating the advantages and disadvantages of employing the rat rather than larger animals such as the dog or pig. As will be seen, many of these are more referable to the small size of the rat rather than to any other particular characteristic.

Advantages of the Rat

1. Closely inbred colonies, which are readily available, may be used, thus reducing variability of behaviour.
2. The use of rats is clearly less expensive than that of larger animals.
3. The small volume of perfusate required makes the use of expensive reagents such as isotopically labelled compounds more economical.
4. The operative procedure in setting up a rat preparation takes no more than 10 minutes, compared with much longer times for the dog. Thus, if a preparation has been for some reason unsatisfactory, it is very practicable to set up a second one.

5. The liver of the rat is divided for the most part into entirely discrete lobes, and thus excision of tissue during the course of an experiment does not give rise to problems of bleeding.
6. A very much larger amount of biochemical information is available for rat liver than for the livers of larger animals. Thus it is more easy to make useful comparisons between results from isolated liver perfusion experiments and those from studies of the liver in intact animals, or of liver slices, homogenates and subcellular fractions.

Disadvantages of the Rat

1. Because of volume consideration, studies on bile are much more practicable in larger animals than in the rat.
2. Studies on hepatic lymph are easier in larger animals, but can be carried out in the rat (Bollman, Cain and Grindlay, 1948).
3. It is difficult to take a large number of liver biopsies in the rat.
4. It is very difficult to perfuse rat liver through the hepatic artery as well as the portal vein. However, the circumstances under which this facility might be important have not been well defined.
5. Studies of perfused livers relevant to hepatic support and transplantation in human liver disease are clearly better done in larger animals.
6. The larger animals can provide their own perfusate.

It should be pointed out that the increasing sensitivity of techniques for estimation of metabolites in tissue has made the sheer bulk of liver tissue in large animals progressively less of an advantage. Finally, the choice of species for any particular investigation may depend on considerations quite different from those enumerated above. If the indirect object of the experiments is to draw conclusions relevant to human physiology or pathology careful consideration should be given to any previous comparative knowledge available in the fields under study; as an example, certain aspects of hepatic gluconeogenesis in the human resemble much more closely the situation in the guinea pig than that in the rat (Söling, Willms and Kleineke, 1971).

It is quite impossible here to review all the variations that have been introduced into the rat perfused liver preparation; these are, in any case, largely dictated by the particular field of study of the individual groups concerned. It will suffice to discuss two of the more recent descriptions (Hems, Ross, Berry and Krebs, 1966; Exton and Park, 1967). These workers developed their preparations from the techniques of Miller, Bly, Watson and Bale (1951) and Mortimore (1961, 1963). The authors have for the past three years used the method of Exton and Park and an account of their slightly modified version of this technique will be given. Hems *et al* (1966) give a particularly detailed description of their preparation; this method will therefore only be outlined briefly.

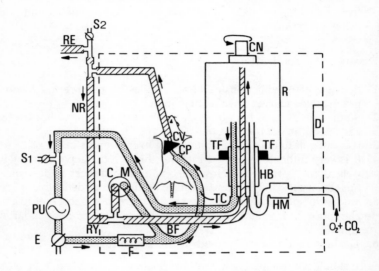

Fig. 34 *Semidiagrammatic view of perfused rat liver preparation from above. The dotted lines indicate the Perspex box. See text for detailed explanation.*

S1, S2, E – sampling ports; RE – medium exit; NR – position of clamp during non-recirculation; PU – pump; RY – re-entry into box; M – manometer; C – chimney; F – filter; BF – bubble trap; TC – thermocouple; CP – portal cannula; CV – venacaval cannula; TF – Teflon seal; HB – hub; CN – centre pin; D – heater; HM – humidifier; R – oxygenator/reservoir.

Technical Description

The Perfusion Circuit (see Figures 34–36)
This is designed to give constant flow through the liver. It is carried out in a Perspex box (42 × 42 × 42 cm), split horizontally into a lid (L) and a lower portion (P). The preparation rests on a Perspex tray (T), resting on rails (RL) (so that it may be moved laterally), at the level of the split. The front face of the lower portion P may be lowered on the hinges (H) so that adjustments to the circuit etc. may be made during the course of the perfusion. The whole box is heated by a fan

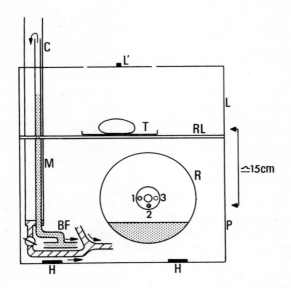

Fig. 35 Semidiagrammatic view of some parts of the circuit seen from the front.
L – lid; L' – subsidiary lid; T – tray; RL – rail; C – chimney; M – manometer; R – oxygenator; P – Perspex box; BF – bubble trap; H – hinges; 1 – medium exit; 2 – medium entry; 3 – gas entry.

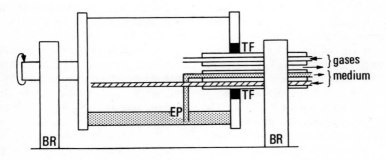

Fig. 36 Semidiagrammatic side view of oxygenator/reservoir.
TF – Teflon seal; BR – brackets; EP – exit point.

and heating element (D) mounted on a lateral wall and controlled by a thermostat usually set at 36°C. Humidification is achieved by a vessel of water on the floor of the box, which has several wide gauze wicks draped over its sides.

The oxygenator and reservoir (R) are combined and the design is almost identical to that shown by Exton and Park (1967) except that the capacity is 4 to 5 times as great, accommodating up to 550 ml of medium. This modification was introduced because we were particularly concerned with non-recirculating perfusions. R consists of a wide tube of Perspex (internal diameter 14 cm, length 15 cm), closed at each end by discs of Perspex. The oxygenator must be fully taken apart for cleaning purposes and the joins between the ends and the tube are rubber O-ring seals, sealing pressure being maintained by suitably placed screws. The proximal end of the oxygenator has a centre hub (HB) which transmits the portal and hepatic venous lines, and the gas mixture. In addition the hub contains an exit for gases, which should be of as large a diameter as possible (e.g. 3–4 mm). The wider this exit, the more protection is provided against build-up of gas pressure in the oxygenator due to inadvertent increases in gas flow; such increase of pressure is transmitted to the venous line and the preparation may be swiftly rendered useless. The hub is rigidly fixed in the bracket (BR) attached to the floor of the box and the oxygenator rotates around it. The seal between the hub and the proximal end is a ring of Teflon (TF) which rotates on the hub with comparatively little friction. The distal end of the oxygenator has a centre pin (CN) coupled to a suitable electric motor, placed outside the box. The oxygenator rotates at 60 rpm and even filming of the perfusate over the whole surface is achieved. Frothing is not a problem. Mixing in the chamber appears to be rapid and is complete within 1 minute. Full studies on the speed of gas equilibration have not been done but we have had no trouble in maintaining steady portal and hepatic venous pH, PCO_2 and PO_2 throughout a perfusion. (Variation of pH < 0.04 units; of PCO_2, < 5 mm Hg; of hepatic venous PO_2 < 6 mm Hg). No systematic trends have been observed in these measurements, and the variations are frequently much less than the above figures. Before the gases enter the oxygenator they are bubbled through water in a humidifier bottle (HM) kept within the box. The gas flow rate is $0.5–1$ l/min. For safety reasons the power supplies to the oxygenator motor and the heater are isolated from the mains by suitable transformers.

Medium from the oxygenator is pumped to the liver by the rotary pump (PU) (Watson Marlow type MHRE) and may be sampled at the point S1. The three-way tap (E) is occasionally useful to evacuate any air which may have inadvertently been allowed to enter at S1. S1, PU and E are actually outside the box. After re-entry at RY the medium passes through a filter (F). This consists of about 2·5 cm of fairly tightly packed glass wool. This filter appears to be essential to maintain a normal appearance of the liver. Exton and Park place a filter within the oxygenator at point EP; we prefer the site F since the filter may be larger here and possibly deals with any red cell fragmentation occurring in the pump. The medium next passes a bubble trap (BF) which is also a side-arm to the manometer (M) and then on to the portal vein cannula. The temperature of the blood entering the liver is monitored by a thermocouple (TC).

Medium leaving the liver through the inferior vena cava first passes to a three-way junction just outside the box. For periods in which the medium recirculates after passage through the liver a clamp is placed on the exit RE. For non-recirculation periods this clamp is transferred to the position NR. Hepatic venous blood may be sampled at the point S2. Measurement of flow rate is achieved by collecting effluent from RE in a graduated cylinder over timed intervals (usually 1 minute). The medium then re-enters the box and passes to the oxygenator, where it drops into the reservoir medium at the opposite end to the point of aspiration of the portal venous medium. At the point of exit into the reservoir, in which the medium is at atmospheric pressure, the end of the venous line is some 12–15 cm below the preparation itself. This prevents swelling of the liver during perfusion (Exton and Park, 1967).

The liver perfusion pressure is measured by the manometer system (M). The contribution of the cannula to the resistance is determined before the preparation is set up by measuring the pressure generated at the proposed flow rate with the portal cannula feeding straight into the venous line. The manometer is contained within a chimney (C) which protrudes through the lid (L). Any overflow from the mano-meter is thus collected and returned to the venous line. The chimney also forms a convenient point at which to fill the circuit.

Cannulae

The cannula (CV) draining the vena cava should be of considerably greater bore than the portal vein cannula (CP). Dimensions of those used by us are as follows: Portal vein cannula ID 0·75 mm, OD, 1·25 mm, length 3·4 cm. Vena cava cannula ID 1·75 mm, OD 2·4 mm, length 2·6 cm. Both are made from stainless steel tubing, are bevelled and have a shallow circular groove ground about 1·5 mm from the tip.

Tubing

The tubing from which the bulk of the circuit is constructed is of opalescent polyvinyl chloride, OD 4 mm, ID 2·9 mm (Portex No. 6, Portland Plastics Limited, Hythe, Kent). With this type of tubing we have found no difference in PCO_2 and PO_2 in medium sampled simultaneously at two points in the circuit some 70 cm apart, with medium flow rate 8 ml/min; in these observations PO_2 was 450 mm Hg and PCO_2 50 mm Hg. Hems *et al* (1966) found it necessary to use glass tubing when gas exchanges were to be measured, since the transparent vinyl tubing usually employed by them was permeable to gases.

The T-junctions and bubble traps are of glass, and it is convenient to use those supplied by the Technicon Instrument Co. for Auto-analyser equipment.

Cleaning of the Apparatus after Use

After use the circuit is completely dismantled and washed through with tap water. It is our practice to discard the Portex tubing after each day's experiment, but many other workers find this unnecessary; the taps, junctions, and oxygenator components are soaked in an alkaline detergent solution (e.g. 'Pyroneg', Diversey Ltd, Barnet, Herts) for about 24 hours. The detergent is then washed out with tap water, then distilled water. When the apparatus is reassembled it is washed out for about 30 min with two changes of 150 ml saline before introduction of the perfusion medium.

Perfusion Medium

Very high flow rates are required to maintain sensitive functions such as gluconeogenesis if the medium does not contain red cells. In the absence of albumin the liver progressively swells. The medium therefore basically contains erythrocytes and albumin in the physio-logical 'saline' solution of Krebs and Henseleit (1932) (referred to as 'buffer' hereafter).

Various sources of erythrocytes have been used by different workers – e.g. rat, bovine (Exton and Park, 1967) expired human red cells (Hems *et al*, 1966) and equine (Cohen *et al*, 1971). Satisfactory perfusions can be obtained with any of these. However, large numbers of rats may have to be sacrificed if homologous cells are insisted upon, and most workers use other sources. The use of expired human cells by Hems *et al* has the advantage of ready availability; furthermore, after 4–5 weeks' storage human cells still have the capacity for oxygen carriage (but see below) but do not glycolyse, this being an advantage if measurements of changes in glucose and lactate concentrations in the medium are being made. However, they have some disadvantages, the most important being that use of human blood must entail a risk of contraction of serum hepatitis by the workers involved. For this reason we abandoned the use of human cells, changing to equine cells. Other perhaps lesser disadvantages of expired cells are the rather greater tendency to haemolysis during perfusion, and the altered oxygen dissociation characteristics due to depletion of 2:3 diphosphoglycerate during storage. Thus, when perfusing with expired cells at a rate of 6–9 ml/min per 100 g total rat weight, at a haematocrit of 20%, hepatic venous PO_2 was quite frequently below 30 mm Hg. With fresh equine cells under the same conditions the PO_2 usually lies between 40 and 50 mm Hg. However, this did not make a significant difference to the rate of gluconeogenesis from lactate, which, as discussed below, is probably a sensitive indicator of the state of the preparation.

400 ml equine blood is taken direct from the donor animal into a standard blood transfusion bottle containing 120 ml acid-citrate-dextrose solution.* The bottle is then stored at 4°C. The cells are satisfactory for at least 10 days after donation. On the day of the perfusion, the cells are spun down, the plasma removed, and the cells washed twice with 2 vols. of saline and twice with 2 vols. buffer. A solution of 4% bovine serum albumin (Armour, Fraction V) in buffer is prepared; cells are then added to it in the proportion of 3 vols. cells to 8 vols. albumin solution. Occasional batches of albumin result in an unsatisfactory appearance of the liver. This may be overcome by dialysis of the 4% albumin solution for 48 hours before use against several changes of buffer. (H.F. Woods, Oxford: personal communication.) The albumin solution is always acid and the pH of the medium as prepared will be low. There is little point in attempting to correct this before the medium has been well circulated and equilibrated (in the absence of the rat) in the perfusion apparatus at the intended temperature and PCO_2 of the experiments. Buffer solution, modified in that the chloride has been replaced by bicarbonate is then added until the pH and PCO_2 are in the desired range (for most applications 7·36–7·42 and 35–42 mm Hg respectively).

*This procedure is kindly performed for us by Wellcome Reagents Ltd., Park Langley Estate, Beckenham, Kent.

The haematocrit, after the addition of solution to adjust the pH, should be between 15 and 21%. Using 94·5% O_2 and 5·5% CO_2 the PO_2 of the medium in the reservoir is usually 400–450 mm Hg. Immediately before preparing the rat, the portal venous and IVC lines, joined together for the preliminary equilibration, are separated, a clamp placed at NR, saline injected at RE to fill the IVC line to the cannula and a second clamp placed at RE.

Operative Technique

At the end of the preparation the liver remains *in situ*, but functionally isolated from the carcass. There is no difficulty in setting up the preparation in animals of weight down to 90g though we have commonly used animals in the weight range 120–150g. The animal, in the dietary state appropriate to the particular study, is anaesthetised by an intraperitoneal injection of sodium pentobarbitone 80 mg/kg and is then weighed. The main lid L is removed from the perfusion apparatus, the rat tray pushed to the right as far as possible, and the subsidiary lid L' placed on the rails to the left of the tray. By this manoeuvre the whole bottom half of the box is thus now again enclosed and fall in temperature of the medium during the setting up of the preparation is minimal. The limbs of the animal are secured to the tray by adhesive tape. The cannulae are inserted into the tubing so that the bevel of the portal vein cannula faces upwards and that of the inferior vena cava (IVC) cannula faces downwards.

A cruciate incision is then made from the symphysis pubis to the xiphisternum, and well into both flanks. The gut is then moved to the left to reveal the posterior abdominal wall. A cotton ligature is passed around the IVC above the R renal vein and a single loop loosely tied (Ligature 1). Heparin, 100 IU, is then injected into the IVC. A second ligature (Ligature 2) is then placed loosely around the portal vein just above the entry of the first major tributary on the left and another about 1 cm lower down (Ligature 3). Any air in the portal venous cannula is carefully expelled. Ligature 3 is tied and used to steady the portal vein. The portal cannula is now either inserted directly into the portal vein, or a small incision made in the vein and the cannula inserted through it. Ligature 2 is now tied in the groove of the portal cannula, the pump switched on, and the IVC immediately cut across with scissors just above its division into the iliac veins. The liver is now being perfused, with no ischaemia time if the cannula has been directly inserted and usually no more than 10 seconds' ischaemia if insertion has been through an incision.

The function of the heart is now irrelevant to the perfusion of the liver. The anterior wall of the rib cage is then widely excised with strong scissors, starting with an upwards incision through the left costal margin. With the left hand the lateral wall of the right atrium is seized with blunt forceps and pulled slightly to the right. This creates a triangular superior surface to the right atrium through which the IVC cannula is thrust, bevel down, into the supra-diaphragmatic portion of the IVC. Because of the negative pressure in this line, it is quite unnecessary to tie this cannula in; once properly inserted it never comes out spontaneously.

The clamp at RE is removed and medium immediately begins to flow into the venous line. Ligature 1 around the abdominal IVC is now tied and the preparation is complete. Medium and blood which have escaped into the tray through the lower IVC incision are wiped away, the subsidiary lid L' removed, the rat tray moved to the centre of the rails and the main and subsidiary lids replaced. After the saline in the IVC line has been expelled and about 5–10 ml of medium has been discarded, the clamp at NR may be shifted to RE if recirculation is required. The flow is adjusted to be between 6 and 7·5 ml/100 g rat weight and is recorded at intervals throughout the experiment, together with observation of temperature and pressure. The whole procedure of setting up the perfusion takes less than 10 minutes. Some workers routinely tie the hepatic artery at the end of the procedure; the value of this manoeuvre has not been established. The bile duct may be cannulated if desired.

Sampling of Liver Tissue during Perfusion

Some care is required in the removal of the left lobe of the liver. The procedure is as follows. A loosely looped ligature is placed round the hilum of the left lobe at the time of setting up the preparation. When the lobe is to be excised the right lobe is gently reflected with a broad spatula. When the ligature is tied a small knob of liver tissue should be included; if this is not done cyanosed blotches may appear in the right lobe, presumably due to distortion of the vascular supply. The ligature is gently pulled moderately tight and in doing so cuts through a small amount of liver tissue; bleeding never seems to occur from this surface, and judged by the cyanosed appearance of the small remnant, it is effectively avascular. The left lobe is then excised with scissors distal to the ligature.

Our observations (Cohen *et al,* 1971) have shown that in Glaxo-Wistar rats the proportion of the total weight of the liver contributed by the left lobe is very constant, whether it is assessed in the starved animal without proceeding to perfusion, or after perfusion. Since this contribution averages 30% it has been our practice to reduce the medium flow rate in proportion after excision of the left lobe.

The Method of Hems et al (1966)

The main differences from the above technique are as follows. Firstly the method of Hems *et al* utilises constant pressure as opposed to a constant volume perfusion. Medium is pumped to the top of a multi-bulb glass oxygenator; gas exchange takes place as the medium flows down the inner surface of the column-like structure and the medium is collected in a reservoir at the foot of the column, from which the liver is directly perfused. The venous effluent from the liver drops into a second reservoir below the animal from which it is pumped to the top of the oxygenator. The rate of pumping of the medium is always more than required to keep the perfusion reservoir level steady and the overflow is diverted directly to the second reservoir. The flow rates employed are higher than in the Exton and Park method (judging from the rat liver weights reported, approximately 10–16 ml/min per 100 g rat) but the haematocrit (approximately 8·5%) is lower.

Criteria of Satisfactory Perfusion

No isolated perfused organ preparation can claim to be 'physiological'. In the absence of controlled delivery to the liver of the full complement of substrates, hormonal and possibly nervous influences, such preparations can only be regarded as models and criteria will be largely tailored to the functions under study. Nevertheless there are certain general criteria which it seems reasonable to employ.

(1) Appearance
The appearance of the perfused liver should be indistinguishable from that of the liver *in situ.* Any blotchiness, however minor, should dictate immediate rejection of that preparation. We have occasionally seen a fine reticular appearance on the surface of the liver, quite distinct from blotchiness; histological examination of such livers suggests that this is due to congestion of subcapsular vessels. Minor

degrees of this probably do not effect the performance of the liver at least in terms of lactate uptake, but any preparation showing this feature more prominently should be rejected.

(2) Absence of Swelling
Exton and Park (1967) demonstrated that the ratio of wet to dry weight is not increased appreciably during perfusion in the preparation above. Hems *et al* (1966) showed that omission of the albumin led to swelling of the liver, but varying the concentration of albumin between 1% and 6% made no difference.

(3) Portal Pressure
In constant volume perfusions we have found the portal pressure usually to be between 12 and 24 cm of medium, depending on the flow. In the majority of preparations the pressure falls slightly but continuously, at least over the first hour. A rise in portal pressure indicates either a block in the circuit or increased hepatic vascular resistance. When the latter is the case the appearance of the liver always becomes unsatisfactory.

(4) Rate of Gluconeogenesis from Lactate
Hems *et al* pointed out that synthetic functions are affected early when a tissue deteriorates, and that gluconeogenesis from lactate was the most exacting synthetic process in terms of requirements for ATP, 6 mols of the nucleotide being required for each mol of glucose formed. The maximal rates of gluconeogenesis from lactate in perfused livers of starved rats found by Hems *et al* and Exton and Park are about 1 μ mol/min/g fresh weight of liver; this value compares favourably with some of those obtained by other workers. We have obtained similar rates in our perfusions. Exton and Park (1969) showed that when the liver was perfused with medium containing lactate, pyruvate, amino-acids and glycerol in the concentrations present *in vivo*, then the rate of gluconeogenesis approached that obtained in starving rats *in vivo*. The somewhat lesser rates *in vitro* might be explicable in terms of the slightly lower temperature of the perfusion compared with the intact animal, and the probable presence *in vivo* of hormones such as glucagon and epinephrine which stimulate gluconeogenesis.

Some differences do however exist between the performances of the two preparations. In the presence of saturating quantities of lactate, no glycogen was formed in the preparation of Hems *et al* after approximately 90 min; small but significant quantities of glycogen were formed after 60 min in the system of Exton and Park (1967).

During maximal gluconeogenesis from lactate no change in adenine nucleotide content of the liver was found by Exton and Park (1969); in contrast, Hems *et al* found a decrease in ATP content and a rise in ADP content. This could be interpreted as indicating better reserves of ATP production in the first method. Against this suggestion, however, is the observation that, in the second method, gluconeogenesis from lactate and urea synthesis from ammonium chloride and ornithine (both processes with high ATP requirements) were able to proceed together at the same maximal rates as observed when the two sets of substances were added singly.

Hems *et al* also investigated the effect of omission of erythrocytes from the perfusate on the rate of glucose formation from lactate; in order to maintain rates similar to those found in their usual preparation the flow had to be increased to above 30 ml/min (liver weight < 5 g).

(5) Oxygen Consumption

Oxygen consumption at maximal rates of gluconeogenesis from lactate was observed to be some 50% higher by Hems *et al* compared with that found by Exton and Park. It is difficult to say whether a higher oxygen consumption is a virtue or not; it is possible that it signifies less efficient use of energy obtained from the oxidation of substrates.

The length of time over which a preparation will function satisfactorily is again dependent on the particular application. Gluconeogenesis from lactate will proceed at full rates for at least 2 hours. Haemolysis during a 2-hour perfusion is slight, especially if fresh erythrocytes are used. The potassium and phosphate contents of the medium rise especially during perfusion. Exton and Park showed that this could be prevented by addition of insulin, 1 mμ/ml of medium; this manoeuvre, however, might be undesirable in some applications.

Choice of Type of Liver Perfusion

This will be dependent on the requirements of the particular study intended. Both the constant volume and constant pressure preparations obviously give satisfactory results according to the above criteria.

Our own view is that, unless it is definitely known that the process under study is not flow dependent at the flows and substrate concentrations to be employed, there is something to be said for using a constant flow method. There is some evidence that hepatic vascular resistance may change during a perfusion, and thus in constant pressure methods flow will also change. If it is intended to calculate uptake or output of substrates and metabolites from the Fick principle, rather than from changes in reservoir concentration, it is advantageous to use slower flow rates and higher haematocrits, to magnify portal-hepatic venous concentration differences as much as possible, whilst maintaining oxygenation. If it is necessary to mini-mise changes imposed by hepatic metabolism on the composition of the perfusate entering the liver, then two options are available – increasing the reservoir volume and using the non-recirculating type of perfusion.

References

Bollman, J.L., Cain, J.C. and Grindlay, J.H. (1948) Techniques for the collection of lymph from the liver, small intestine or thoracic duct of the rat. *J. Lab. Clin. Med.* **33,** 1349.

Cohen, R.D., Iles, R.A., Barnett, D., Howell, M.E.O. and Strunin, J. (1971) The effect of changes in lactate uptake on the intracellular pH of the perfused rat liver. *Clin. Sci.* **41,** 159.

Corey, E.L. and Britton, S.W. (1941) Glycogen levels in the isolated liver perfused with cortico-adrenal extract, insulin and other prepara-tions. *Am. J. Physiol.* **131,** 783.

Exton, J.H. and Park, C.R. (1967) Control of gluconeogenesis in liver, I, General features of gluconeogenesis in the perfused livers of rats. *J. Biol. Chem.* **242,** 2622.

Exton, J.H. and Park, C.R. (1969) Control of gluconeogenesis in liver, III, Effects of L-lactate, pyruvate, fructose, glucagon, epinephrine and adenosine 3'5' – monophosphate on gluconeogenic intermediates in the perfused rat liver. *J. Biol. Chem.* **244,** 1424.

Hems, R., Ross, B.D., Berry, M.N. and Krebs, H.A. (1966) Gluconeogenesis in the perfused rat liver. *Biochem. J.* **101,** 284.

Miller, L.L., Bly, C.G., Watson, M.L. and Bale, W.F. (1951) The dominant role of the liver in plasma protein synthesis. A direct study of the isolated perfused rat liver with the aid of lysine – C^{14}. *J. Experimen. Med.* **94,** 431.

Mortimore, G.E. (1961) Effect of insulin on potassium transfer in isolated rat liver. *Am. J. Physiol.* **200,** 1315.

Mortimore, G.E. (1963) Effect of insulin on release of glucose and urea by isolated rat liver. *Am. J. Physiol.* **204,** 699.

Söling, H.D., Willms, B. and Kleineke, J. (1971) Regulations of gluconeogenesis in rat and guinea pig livers. *Regulation of Gluconeogenesis*. Ed. Söling, H.D. and Willms, B. Academic Press and Georg Thieme Verlag, New York and Stuttgart, pp. 210–226.

CHAPTER NINE

Stomach

Perfusion of the Isolated Canine Stomach

Review of the Literature

Some of the earliest observations on the isolated stomach were made by Lim *et al* (1927) (i) firstly upon the transplanted stomach and later on the isolated preparation cross-circulated with another dog (1927) (ii). In these latter studies perfusion was established only after an anoxic period of ten to fifteen minutes. It was noted that although the stomach would secrete acid in response to histamine, it failed to respond to feeding of the perfusing animal although a Heidenhain pouch in the same animal gave a good response to the meal. It was not regarded therefore as a useful test object for the humoral mechanism of gastric secretion. Further studies were carried out however and a later communication from the same group (1927) (iii) describes extensive investigations into the vaso-motor responses of this extrinsically denervated preparation.

Moody *et al* (1962) developed a gastric wedge preparation which was perfused initially from the animal by the short gastric vessels, but which could then be transferred gradually to a pump-oxygenator system. This method had the advantage of avoiding any period of anoxia during the transition to isolated perfusion. Salmon and Assimacopoulos (1964) described an isolated stomach preparation which was perfused with a roller pump, using blood oxygenated with the donor dog's own lung. They reported acid secretion in response to histamine in only 30% of their preparations. Failure to secrete was believed to be due in some instances to prolonged periods of ischaemia before perfusion via the circuit was re-established, and also to the use of homologous donor blood. The presence of some motor activity in these preparations was noted but no detailed studies were reported. Dritsas and Kowalewski (1966) developed a stomach preparation which was cross-circulated, after an anoxic period of 5-10 minutes, with another dog; sustained acid secretion was observed in response to intra-arterial histamine. However, no reports were made on the motility of the preparation. Blood flow measurements were not given in absolute values by either of these two groups of workers, although Salmon and Assimacopoulos reported perfusion pressures of 60-140 mm Hg. They also noted that over-perfusion rapidly led to oedema of the preparation.

Way and Hawley (1969) using a very sophisticated perfusion system of membrane oxygenator and pulsatile arterial pump were still unable to avoid the initial period of anoxia in setting up the preparation. They reported data on acid secretion, electrolyte changes, sugar metabolism and oxygen consumption by the preparation, but did not use the preparation for anything other than secretory studies. A comparison of secretion, in the cross-circulated, and the isolated perfused, stomach preparation has recently come from Canada in a paper by Kowalewski and Scharf (1971).

A method has been developed in this laboratory for perfusion of the isolated canine stomach, using the dog's own heparinised blood, which avoids any initial period of anoxia, during the setting up of the preparation (Green and Hardcastle, 1970). The stomach may be perfused alone, or together with the lower oesophagus and duodenum, making it possible to perform a variety of studies on the gastro-oesophageal sphincter, the pylorus and the biliary sphincter. Previous workers have concentrated mainly upon the secretory aspect of the perfused stomach. Studies on motility and myoelectrical activity would appear to have been confined to the muscle strip, or whole-animal preparations. However this type of work has been found to be readily extended to include observations on the isolated perfused stomach, and some of the data on motility (Green, Hardcastle and Ritchie, 1970) and myoelectrical activity (Green and Hardcastle, 1970) have already been reported.

A detailed method for setting up the preparation, and its behaviour under basal conditions are described in this and the following section. The stability and reproducibility of the functional aspects of the oesophagus, stomach and duodenum will be described and an assessment made of the value of the preparation for physiologic studies.

The Perfusion Circuit and its Operation

The Apparatus

The pump-oxygenator system, water bath and organ chamber are mounted on a single, mobile trolley, the level of which is below that of the operating table. As there is no pump in the venous side of the system, it is important that the oxygenator itself should be five or so centimetres below the organ chamber to allow free drainage of blood from the preparation. The venous pressure may then be controlled by simple alteration of the resistance to flow in the line itself. For perfusion rates of up to 400 cc/min this system of drainage is adequate and has the advantage of simplicity.

The basic circuit is shown in Figure 37, and is the one used for the majority of perfusion experiments. Alternative configurations are discussed later in this section. All tubing is medical grade soft PVC with an internal diameter of 5 mm and we have found this sufficiently non-toxic for routine use. As an alternative, Silicone rubber tubing of the same size may be used, with the disadvantage of a considerable increase in the cost. The arterial cannula is rigid PVC tubing of the same grade, and must be sufficiently long to permit entry into the aorta via the femoral artery. A heating coil is incorporated in the arterial line and is maintained in the water bath at 37°C.

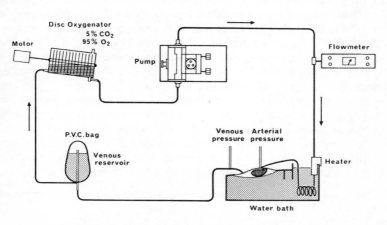

Fig. 37 The perfusion circuit used in isolated stomach perfusion.

A 6-inch polycarbonate disc oxygenator* has been found most satisfactory. It is easily dismantled for cleaning, and is the only part of the circuit which is re-used. With a disc rotation of 60 rpm satisfactory oxygenation is achieved with flows of up to 300 cc/min, which is well in excess of the range encountered in stomach perfusion work. The blood is supplied to the arterial line by an occlusive roller+ or a pulsatile pump. Stopcocks are placed in the circuit, close to the preparation for injection of drugs and obtaining blood samples for analysis. Perfusion pressure is measured by a line placed in the aorta and connected to a strain gauge transducer. Venous pressure is measured by a side-arm to the cannula within the superior mesenteric vein itself.

The water bath (Figure 38) serves also as the base of the organ chamber. The perfused organ rests on a thin sheet of polythene stretched across the water surface, and is covered with a second sheet before being totally enclosed by a Perspex cover. This provides a soft, mobile bed, and simulates the intra-abdominal cavity. Perfusion and monitoring lines are led to the preparation via small slots let into the sides of the organ chamber, which itself slopes upward at 5° to allow the free drainage of gastric secretions.

Mode of Operation

The circuit is primed with normal saline from a Steriflex‡ litre pack, which then serves as the venous reservoir. The arterial and venous lines are joined together and the saline is circulated for 15 minutes to ensure that the system is free from trapped air bubbles. A modified cleaning régime using two saline washes is recommended. The final wash is then discarded, leaving only a sufficient volume to prime the bottom of the oxygenator, the pump and the arterial line. Blood from the donor animal is run into the reservoir from the superior mesenteric vein, and when this has been fully oxygenated, it is pumped into the arterial line to displace the saline. With 250 cc of blood the perfusion may be initiated, and as the animal is bled the system is filled to its capacity of 2,000 cc. One or two points about the technique of running the perfusion, particularly during the early stages, are worthy of note.

It is important to watch the level of blood in the oxygenator; if this is allowed to fall too low the pump will suck air and the preparation will be ruined. There are a number of small vessels that are untied

---

*Cardiovascular Electrodynamics Corporation, 537, Stanford Road, Baltimore 29, Maryland, U.S.A.

+ Flow Inducer M.H.R.E. Mk. III, Watson Marlow Limited, Falmouth, Cornwall.

‡ Allen & Hanburys Limited, London, E.2. England

when perfusion is first established and some blood is inevitably lost until they are secured. It is for this reason that the level in the oxygenator may fall, and conversely, as they are tied off, the peripheral resistance to the pump will rise and flow must be turned down to maintain a constant perfusion pressure of 60 mm Hg. It is during this final period of the operative procedure that obstruction to the venous return may occur and the person in charge of the perfusion should be on the alert for this complication. Any fall in the amount of blood in the system at this stage suggests obstruction to the venous outflow and should be brought to the attention of the operator. Venous engorgement leads to a rapid and irreversible deterioration in the preparation.

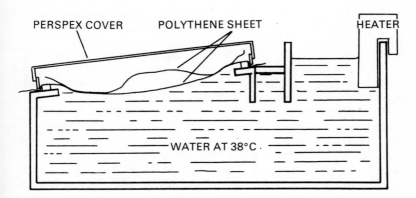

Fig. 38 Organ chamber incorporated into a water bath. The preparation is sandwiched between two thin sheets of polythene and rests on the surface of the water.

As the circuit is filled with blood the height of the reservoir should be adjusted to maintain the level of blood in the oxygenator just below the spindle. If it is allowed to go higher than this the area exposed to the gas mixture becomes less and less and the efficiency falls off. If, on the other hand, the level is allowed to fall, the discs cut the surface of the blood more and more obliquely and this quickly leads to foaming with an increase in the amount of damage to red cells and plasma proteins.

Once all the blood has been added to the circuit, samples should be taken for arterial and venous pH, pCO_2 and pO_2 determination. This provides a check not only on the oxygenating system, but also on whether the organ is being adequately perfused. A venous oxygen saturation of less than 50% strongly suggests underperfusion and it should be corrected at this stage. This situation may easily arise during the first 30 minutes particularly if the perfusion is controlled on the basis of pressure in the absence of any direct measurement of flow. Blood obtained by total exsanguination is known to contain large amounts of catecholamines (Miller and Bentley, 1958) and this is reflected by a rise in perfusion pressure as the last of the blood is added to the circuit, often in the order of 30–40 mm Hg. This effect is short-lived and it would appear that passage of the blood through the stomach preparation leads to inactivation of these vaso-active substances for within 15 minutes the perfusion pressure will usually return to its previous level. For this reason we have found it essential to use calibrated pumps, or to incorporate in the circuit an electromagnetic flow probe. Adequacy of perfusion must be based on accurate measurement of blood flow and not perfusion pressure.

Alternative Perfusion Circuits

Membrane oxygenators In Figure 39 is shown a circuit for use with small membrane oxygenators. As before we have not used a pump on the venous side, and therefore to avoid a negative pressure in the mesenteric vein we have incorporated two reservoirs. Blood drains from the preparation to reservoir 1 and then by gravity through the oxygenator to reservoir 2. This arrangement will permit flows of up to 200 cc/min using undiluted blood. For higher flow rates than this the resistance within the oxygenator is too great and it becomes necessary to pump the blood from one reservoir to the other. We have used this circuit with the Lande-Edwards 1 sq. metre unit*, and with the oxygenator unit developed by Travenol Laboratories† for organ preservation. Satisfactory gas exchange has been obtained with flow rates of up to 400 cc/min, and there is significantly less damage to the red cells as judged by measurement of free haemoglobin in the plasma. Both units are currently available from the manufacturers, and are regarded as an improvement in the technique of organ perfusion. Their great disadvantage is the high cost, as the units are disposable and cannot be used again.

Cross-Perfusion Figure 40 shows the circuit used when the experimental protocol requires the presence of a second animal to provide oxygenated blood. In this situation while on cross-perfusion, the oxygenator is not in use and merely acts as a reservoir for blood from the animal which is then pumped to the stomach under the same

---

* Edwards Laboratories, Santa Ana, Palo Alto, California.

† Travenol Laboratories Inc. (Artificial Organs Division), Morton Grove, Illinois, 60053, U.S.A.

controlled conditions of flow and pressure as before. The donor animal is kept anaesthetised and ventilated with oxygen, and heparin 5,000 units is administered hourly. The outflow of blood from the animal is matched to the demands of the pump by partial occlusion of the cannula in the femoral artery. By turning on the oxygenator, and transferring the clamp at position A to B, and the clamp at position C

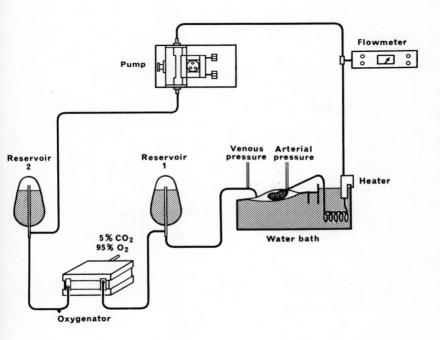

Fig. 39 A diagram showing the perfusion circuit when a membrane oxygenator is used. Note reservoir 1 which acts as a gravity feed for the oxygenator.

to D it is possible to transfer the stomach from a state of cross-perfusion to isolated perfusion. The perfusing dog tolerates this procedure very well and we have been able to conduct experiments for up to 6 hours in duration. After prolonged anaesthesis a metabolic acidosis often develops but this is easily corrected with an intravenous infusion of 0·6 m Sodium Lactate or administration of the buffer tris hydro amino methanol (THAM).

General Remarks about Stomach Perfusions

Arterial Blood Supply

The oesophagus and stomach are perfused through the coeliac axis:
if the total length of the duodenum is also required then perfusion via
the inferior pancreatico-duodenal branch of the superior mesenteric
artery has to be included.

The arterial cannula is placed in a segment of aorta at the level of
the above branches. An aortic segment is used, rather than directly
cannulating the coeliac and superior mesenteric arteries, for several
reasons. Firstly, it is technically much easier to do it this way,

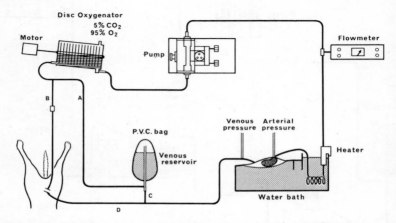

Fig. 40 A diagram showing the circuits used for cross-perfusion and its transferal to isolated perfusion. Note that the venous reservoir is excluded from the circuit when the stomach is being cross-perfused.

because both the coeliac and superior mesenteric arteries are relatively inaccessible for direct cannulation. Secondly, if the direct
method is used then a period of anoxia, however short, cannot be
avoided. It will be realised from reviewing the literature that an anoxic
period has been included in the majority of previous attempts at
isolated stomach perfusions. Thirdly, the inherent elasticity of the
aortic segment is used to protect the smaller calibre fore- and mid-gut
vessels from the full force of the pump's pulsatile input.

The operation is so designed that those branches of the coeliac and
superior mesenteric arteries which are not essential for perfusion are
excluded. The hepatic and splenic arteries are tied off as near the liver

and spleen as possible. Unless this is done damage to the gastro-duodenal and short gastric vessels will occur. If the duodenum is to be included then the superior mesenteric artery is tied beyond the origin of the inferior pancreatico-duodenal. In oesophageal perfusions, the blood supply relies on the oesophageal branch of the left gastric artery. It is not possible to preserve an oesophageal blood supply directly from the aortic segment because of troublesome blood loss. An arteriogram of the isolated stomach and duodenum is shown in Figure 41.

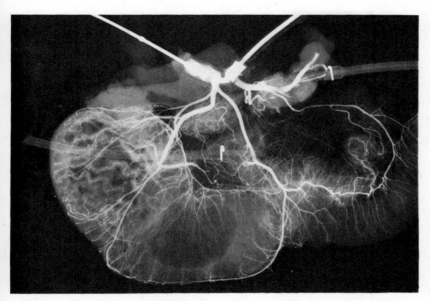

Fig. 41 An arteriogram of the isolated stomach and duodenum is shown. Note the short cuff of aorta at the top with filling of the coeliac axis on the left and the superior mesenteric artery on the right.

Venous Drainage

All venous drainage, including the lower part of the oesophagus, is via the portal venous system. The venous cannula is positioned in the superior mesenteric vein so that its tip lies at its junction with the splenic vein. The one exception is if the whole of the duodenum is included, when the tip is positioned below the entry of the inferior pancreatico-duodenal vein into the superior mesenteric vein. The absence of venous valves enables the venous blood to drain retrogradely. This avoids cannulating the portal vein at the porta hepatis which is technically more difficult. Earlier perfusion did include a Y-shaped venous line when both the portal vein at the porta hepatis and the superior mesenteric vein below were cannulated. This is now thought to be unnecessary as adequate venous drainage can be obtained with the one cannula placed in the superior mesenteric vein.

Bleeding Lines
Blood losses at the time of operation and from the isolated organ are unavoidable. The amounts vary and obviously they decrease as operative experience increases. However, it is important to prime the perfusion circuit with as much blood as possible in order to prepare for loss from the isolated preparation, and to avoid excess recirculation, which would occur with a small circuit volume. The latter, because of increased contact with the pump and oxygenator, will result in an increased haemolysis rate. A system of bleeding cannulae is used which provides the maximum amount of blood with which to prime the circuit. The major volume is drained directly into the circuit from either the venous cannula in the superior mesenteric vein or from the arterial cannula in the aorta. The remainder is obtained from cannulae in the common carotid artery and in the inferior vena cava. If the circulating volume is small then the blood collected from these can be infused into the circuit via the oxygenator. It is however wise to avoid infusing the last 100–200 cc of blood from the inferior vena cava because of its high catecholamine content.

Preparation of the Animal
It is essential that the animal should be in the laboratory kennels for several days prior to surgery, firstly to ensure that it is in good condition, with particular attention given to the nutritional state, and secondly to allow adequate dietary preparation to ensure an empty stomach on the day of operation. We have found that a liquid diet of Complan and milk given for two days is adequate. On the morning of operation the dog should be walked and encouraged to empty its colon and bladder.

Surgical Procedure

After induction of anaesthesia with intravenous sodium thiopentone 50 mg/kg, the animal is placed in the supine position upon the operating table and tied securely. A diathermy pad should be sited under the neck. Ventilation with oxygen is maintained via an endotracheal tube, which should be cuffed to avoid insufflation of the stomach. The common femoral artery and vein in the left groin are exposed, and tapes placed around the vessels in readiness for cannulation later. The carotid arteries in the neck are prepared in a similar way. The abdomen should now be opened by a long mid-line incision extending from the xiphoid to a point 5 centimetres below the umbilicus. All bleeding vessels are carefully controlled with diathermy before placing two hook retractors just below the costal margins and securing these laterally to the sides of the operating table.

This positioning of the two retractors creates a diamond shaped exposure of the upper abdomen which is adequate for all the subsequent dissection prior to the commencement of perfusion. Gentle traction on the spleen permits inspection of the stomach, and it should be very gently palpated to ensure that it is empty. It should not be seen or handled again until perfusion has been established. The subsequent dissection is directed towards isolation of the tissue to be perfused and preparation of the appropriate vessels for cannulation. It may conveniently be described in three stages.

1. Exposure of the superior mesenteric vein.
2. Resection of the intestine not to be included in the perfusion.
3. Exposure of the aorta at the level of the coeliac axis.

Exposure of the Superior Mesenteric Vein
The caecum and the colon are held up by an assistant, and the peritoneal fold behind the duodenal-jejunal flexure is divided close to the bowel, where it will be found to be quite avascular. Attention is now directed to the adhesion of the mesoduodenum to the ileo-caecal region. With the scissors, an avascular plane may be entered, close to the wall of the caecum, which leads directly down to the superior mesenteric vein. It is better to continue down with the nose of the scissors rather than using finger or gauze dissection as this may lead to bleeding from small vessels with staining of the surrounding tissues. There will always be found, in relation to the inferior pancreatico-duodenal vessels, a lymph node; if enlarged its vascular supply should be coagulated with diathermy. The exposed vein is gently cleared, and tapes placed around it, 2 centimetres below the inferior pancreatico-duodenal vein. If the duodenum is to be included in the preparation the superior mesenteric artery, which will be found sometimes to the left, sometimes behind, but always intimately related to the vein, is ligated in continuity distal to the origin of the inferior pancreatico-duodenal vessel. If the stomach alone is to be perfused the superior mesenteric artery is ligated flush with the aorta. This step is essential

to ensure that no bleeding occurs from the pedicle containing the prepared superior mesenteric vein.

Resection of the Intestine

All the intestine distal to the part to be perfused is now resected. If the stomach alone is required, the duodenum and pancreas are divided 1 to 2 centimetres beyond the pylorus. It is advisable to ligate the superior pancreatico-duodenal vessels behind the first part of the duodenum as they descend from the free edge of lesser omentum. Once this has been done the duodenum should be transected first, retaining the proximal cut end in a clamp, as this may be opened later to gain access to the stomach. The pancreas is divided next at the same level, the proximal end being carefully tied with a soft tape to avoid cutting through this delicate tissue; troublesome bleeding from pancreatic veins always occurs if this is allowed to happen. Alternatively the whole pancreas may be dissected off from below the greater curvature, great care being taken to tie off the small vessels supplying the gland from the splenic artery. If the duodenum is to be included in the preparation, then division of the bowel is performed below the inferior pancreatico-duodenal vessels, and in this case the preparation usually includes the whole of the pancreas. Once this division has been made, the blood supply to the small bowel is divided between ligatures working down the branches as they come off the superior mesenteric vessels, as far as the site in the vein selected for cannulation.

At this level it will be seen that the remaining small bowel, and the colon, may be easily removed en bloc and a stout ligature around the superior mesenteric vein and its associated lymph node completes the preparation of the vascular pedicle. If this is cut long and marked with an artery forceps subsequent cannulation is greatly facilitated. Division of the inferior mesenteric artery and the rectum allows the unwanted bowel to be removed from the animal.

Exposure of the Aorta

Careful retraction by an assistant is the key to this next part of the operation. With one hand the spleen is displaced upwards and towards the liver. In this way any possible trauma to the stomach is avoided. With the other hand the left kidney is gently displaced in a downward direction. The aorta, coeliac axis, superior mesenteric and renal arteries are clearly visible. The peritoneum is incised, commencing near the renal artery, in an upward and lateral direction across the large lumbar artery and vein which are clearly visible. There are usually a number of very small vessels and these should be coagulated with diathermy. The aorta will now be visible and a tape is placed around it, between the renal and superior mesenteric arteries. It is fortunate that just here there are no lumbar vessels and a right-angled clamp may safely be passed behind the aorta to facilitate the passage of the tape which is going to be used later to tie the perfusion cannula in place. Finally the large lumbar artery and vein are ligated in continuity, as is a smaller artery which will be seen coursing upwards along the left diaphragmatic crus.

Preparation for Perfusion

The animal is anticoagulated with 10,000 units of heparin and after a period of two minutes to allow for adequate circulation the cannulae are placed in the following order.

The venous line is placed in the superior mesenteric vein and tied securely to the pedicle noting, and preferably marking, the position in which it lies in order to avoid the risk of an unnoticed twist later on, with venous outflow obstruction and almost certain irreversible damage to the preparation. The clamp is removed from the line and blood is allowed to flow into the venous reservoir. It may take five minutes before sufficient blood has entered the oxygenator to prime the arterial line and during this time bleeding cannulae are placed in the carotid arteries and in the inferior vena cava via the femoral vein.

Finally the arterial line, primed with oxygenated blood and free from bubbles, is passed up into the aorta via the left common femoral artery. A little paraffin on the cannula smoothes its introduction into the rather narrow external iliac artery, but once this has been negotiated, the tip may, by palpation, be accurately sited at the level of the coeliac axis. The tape above the renal artery is now tied securely around the cannula.

Institution of Perfusion

At this stage, before describing the final surgical procedure, there are several points about the technique that are worthy of note. Firstly, at no time has the stomach been deprived of its blood supply, and at this stage is still being perfused by the animal's own heart. Later, as the animal is bled and the cardiac output falls, perfusion is smoothly taken over by the arterial pump. Secondly, the venous drainage from the stomach may go in two directions: via the venous line to the circuit, or via the portal vein and the liver to the inferior vena cava, where we have previously sited a bleeding cannula. There is therefore, at this stage, an alternative route for the blood to take should the venous line become twisted or kinked. Thirdly, the spleen has not yet been tied off, and this is important because it may contain 500–600 cc of blood which is required for the perfusion circuit. As bleeding progresses it will be observed to contract and at that stage it may be excluded from the circuit.

Final Dissection

The chest is opened by a median sternotomy, and the chest walls retracted well laterally with the hooks. The diaphragm is divided at its origin and the phrenic nerves cut to prevent it from twitching. The carotid and I.V.C. lines are allowed to drain into heparinised bottles. The blood pressure in the arterial line is noted continuously and will be seen to fall as the heart fails. At 80 mm Hg perfusion is commenced from the circuit and the aorta cross-clamped above the diaphragm. A second clamp is placed across the porta hepatis having ensured that the venous line is lying straight and untwisted. The preparation is now perfused totally from the perfusion apparatus.

It is necessary now to tie off the remaining lumbar arteries and this may be done from the left side of the aorta, rolling it over to allow access to those on the right. It is of particular importance to secure the vessel that runs up the right crus to supply the diaphragm. The aorta is transected above the aortic clamp, and while occluding it lower down near the cannula tip, a tap is tied into the top end which later allows blood to be sampled and arterial pressure to be measured. It is important to have 2 to 3 centimetres of aorta above the cannula as this provides the elastic compliance that contributes to the pulsatile wave form, and protects the micro-circulation of the stomach from the direct force of the arterial pump. The aorta below the tie around the cannula is separated from the I.V.C. and the left kidney is removed. It is also important to divide the origin of the right crus. If the stomach alone is to be perfused, the oesophagus is divided above the diaphragm, preserving carefully the vagus nerves if desired. Inclusion of the oesophagus in the preparation is described at the end of this section.

At this stage the splenic vessels should be ligated, particular care being taken to preserve the short gastric vessels which arise very near the hilum at its upper end. We have found it convenient to leave the spleen attached but excluded from the perfusion as it provides some protection and support for the stomach. Attention is finally directed to the right side of the aorta. The vessels at the porta hepatis are detached from the liver and simply tied off. Before doing so however it is important to look behind the free edge of lesser omentum as sometimes the gastro-duodenal artery may originate high up near the porta. The lesser omentum is separated all the way up to the right triangular ligament and the small vessels contained within it ligated. It will be found that a finger may now be passed down behind the diaphragm between the aorta and the I.V.C. in the right para vertebral gutter. Using this as a guide the numerous vasa vasorum that pass laterally from the aorta to supply the I.V.C. are secured with several stout ligatures. Once this has been done the I.V.C., and, higher up, the diaphragm may be divided and no bleeding will occur.

This frees the stomach from the liver, right kidney and adrenal gland. Finally the arterial cannula is dissected out from the left groin, and the preparation is ready to be transferred to the organ chamber.

Inclusion of the Oesophagus

In preparing for gastro-oesophageal perfusion, the oesophagus will at this stage have remained untouched. It is isolated in the following way. The vessels coming off the arch of the aorta, and the trachea, are divided. The arch itself is also divided as it passes backwards and to the left of the oesophagus. Division of the anterior meso-oesophagus allows the heart and lungs to be removed, revealing the entire oesophagus lying in the posterior mediastinum and attached to the chest wall by its dorsal mesentery. It is then divided at the level of the aortic arch, and the mesentery itself freed from the chest wall by cutting with the diathermy as far away from the oesophagus as possible to avoid damage to the left vagus nerve. Bleeding from this cut edge is however often a problem, although its presence reflects good perfusion of the oesophagus itself. It may be necessary to oversew this edge with a continuous silk or catgut suture. The oesophagus is now quite free, and the preparation ready for transfer to the organ chamber.

Transferring the Preparation to the Perfusion Chamber

Two people are needed to transfer the organ from the dog to the perfusion chamber. The operator is responsible for lifting the preparation and maintaining its anatomy as near normal as possible. The assistant ensures that the arterial and venous lines do not come under any tension.

The organ is placed on the water cushion with both the arterial and venous lines lying underneath the preparation. The arterial line usually lies satisfactorily, but the venous line, with its more mobile pedicle, can become twisted. If venous obstruction occurs the top end of the portal vein becomes distended. Once in position it is advisable that the perfusion lines should be fixed with adhesive tape to avoid the risk of kinking and traction on the cannulae. The venous return should be checked at this stage.

In preparations which include a length of duodenum it is wise to insert a wide fenestrated polythene tube into the cut end of the duodenum to prevent the accumulation of secretions.

If the oesophagus is included, its cut ends should be fixed to the rim of the perfusion chamber by means of two silk ligatures in such a way as to maintain an acute gastro-oesophageal angle.

The preparations are then douched with warm saline solution and covered with a sheet of polythene.

Assessment of the Perfused Oesophagus, Stomach and Duodenum

This assessment covers the first three hours of perfusion only and shows that for this period of time the preparation behaves in a predictable and reproducible fashion and lends itself as a model for physiologic studies on a truly isolated organ.

After this period, however, certain features appear which suggest a deleterious effect of the perfusion system on the preparation. The omentum becomes glassy and oedematous, petechial haemorrhages appear on the pancreas and the exocrine secretion becomes tinged with blood. The spontaneous motility exhibited early on becomes less vigorous and eventually disappears.

Electrodes monitoring the gastric pacemaker in time indicate its failure by a slowing of rate and irregularity of rhythm. After many hours it may completely disappear, as may the transmucosal potential difference. These changes, however, do take time: up to six hours and sometimes longer.

The one exception appears to be in the gastro-oesophageal and pyloric sphincter areas. Sphincteric function seems to deteriorate more quickly. After two hours the gastro-oesophageal sphincter pressure slowly begins to decrease and is associated with a reduction in the amplitude of the electrical recordings.

The assessment of the preparation may be considered under four general headings:

1. Biochemical parameters
2. Electrical activity
3. Mechanical activity
4. Secretion

The first of these is common to all the preparations described in this chapter. The others are more conveniently discussed under the headings Stomach and Duodenum and Gastro-oesophageal Junction.

Biochemical Parameters

The monitoring of routine biochemical parameters with regard to all isolated perfusions has been dealt with in the general section of this book. Included here are certain observations which are pertinent to the oesophageal, gastric and duodenal perfusions. These are shown in Figures 42a–f. They cover the first three hours of perfusion and demonstrate some stability in the system during the early period when the preparation is considered to be of most value for study. All electrolytes, pH and blood gas tensions are maintained within acceptable limits. The plasma proteins show no change either in total values or in the A/G ratio which suggests that there is no significant destruction of these by the oxygenator.

It is interesting to note that there is a steady fall of blood sugar, indicative of uptake and utilisation by the preparation. For this reason we have adopted a policy of routine addition of glucose, at hourly intervals, to the perfusate in sufficient quantity to maintain a blood sugar level of 100 mg%. We believe the stability and reproducibility of these basic parameters to be an essential feature of the perfusion, and any preparation which does not behave in this way should be regarded as unsuitable for study.

Stomach and Duodenum

Electrical Activity

The original work of Alvarez and Mahoney (1922) drew attention to the presence of a recurring electrical potential which could be detected by an electrode placed on the serosal surface of a viscus. Since then advances in amplification and recording techniques have led to a more precise analysis of the electrical activity of smooth muscle, in particular to distinguish between a slow, or primary wave,

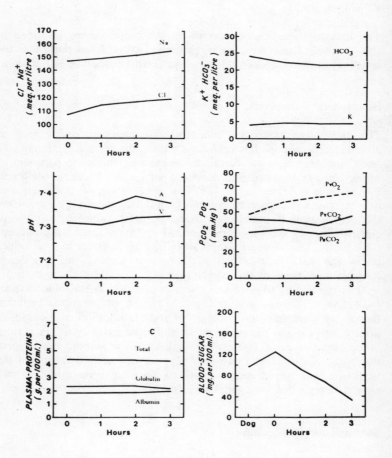

Fig. 42 Figures (a) – (f) demonstrate the stability of the electrolytes, pH, blood gases and plasma proteins during the first three hours of perfusion. Figure (f) demonstrates the changes seen in the blood sugar level when no sugar has been added to the circuit.

and faster spike activity. The slow wave, sometimes referred to as the primary wave, basic electrical rhythm, or pace-setter potential, is omnipresent, and may be detected in the presence or absence of any motor activity. Spike potentials are recorded only in the presence of motor activity and when present they occur after the slow wave. The slow wave, therefore, sets the maximum frequency at which the viscus will contract.

A remarkably constant slow wave recurring at a frequency of 5/min has been described in the intact canine stomach by Kelly, Code and Elveback (1969). It was believed to originate high in the body of the stomach, and has been shown to be propagated aborally, with increasing velocity, to the pylorus. In contrast, the duodenal slow wave described by Hermon-Taylor and Code (1971) has a frequency of 18–19/min. An investigation into the relationship between antral and duodenal electrical activity by Allen, Poole and Code (1964) has shown that the gastric and duodenal slow waves occur quite independently.

Method of Study

For a description of the methodology of electrical recordings in smooth muscle the reader is referred to the review by Daniel and Chapman (1963).

We have preferred the method of bipolar recording, with silver/-silver chloride electrodes (Figure 43) placed on the serosal surface of the stomach and duodenum with fine silk sutures. Amplifiers with a frequency response from d.c. to 700 Hz run at a time constant of 1·2 seconds, coupled to a Mingograf 81 ink-jet recorder have been used.

Electrical Activity of the Unstimulated Preparation

The Stomach

The gastric slow wave recurs at a frequency of 4·8–5·2 per minute and is of greater amplitude in the antrum than in the body of the stomach. In all preparations there was a distinct level above which no activity could be recorded (Figure 44). Serial electrodes placed distally from this point, however, show clearly the increasing amplitude of the slow wave, and also its orderly propagation toward the pylorus (Figure 45). If the speed of propagation between electrodes is measured, it will be found to increase as the slow wave sweeps through the antrum (Figure 46). All the preparations exhibit vigorous spontaneous motility, and this is associated with the occurrence of spike potentials following every slow wave (Figure 47). There is thus a propagated wave of contraction which passes down the stomach to the pylorus, and in this isolated preparation its frequency is that of the slow wave.

The Duodenum

Slow wave activity is recorded at a frequency of 17–19 per minute in the duodenum, which, like the stomach, exhibits spontaneous motility at the frequency of the slow wave. The associated spike potentials are clearly seen (Figure 47). Propagation of the slow wave is seldom seen in the isolated duodenum. However, when it occurs the velocity of propagation is between 6–8 cm/sec. More often, multiple electrodes record uncoordinated electrical activity, and the duodenum will exhibit rhythmic segmentation but not waves of peristalsis.

These observations on the isolated perfused stomach are comparable with findings in the whole animal although there are some small but interesting differences. The frequency of the pace-setter potential varies little from the observations of many workers. However, its

Fig. 43 The electrodes are silver/silver chloride, two millimetres in length, mounted on Perspex. They are placed on the serosal surface of the stomach with fine silk sutures.

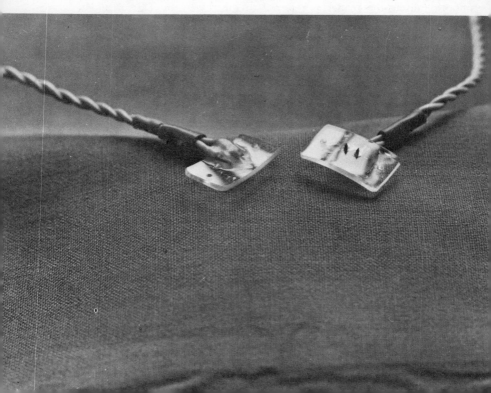

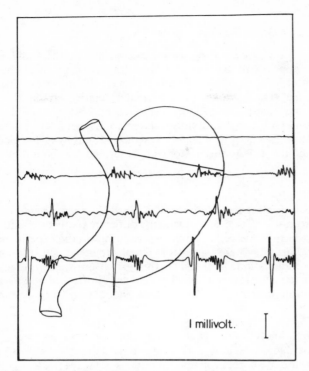

Fig. 44 *The pacesetter potential recorded from the body and antrum of the stomach are shown. Note the greater amplitude in the antrum. The line drawn between the greater and lesser curvatures delineates that part of the stomach from which no pacemacer activity can be recorded.*

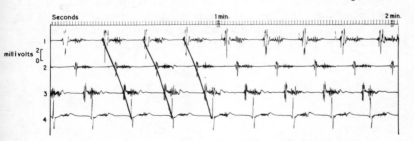

Fig. 45 *The orderly propagation of the pacesetter potential from electrode 1 on the body of the stomach to electrode 4 on the antrum is demonstrated by the lines linking three successive cycles. In this preparation the amplitude of the potential in electrode 1 was unusually large.*

origin or, conversely, disappearance high up in the body of the stomach appears to be different from the concept of Weber and Kohatsu (1970) who placed this crucial region more distinctly towards the greater curvature. Of greater interest still is the spontaneous and continuous motility exhibited by both the stomach and duodenum, and this is possibly related to its complete autonomic denervation. Certainly it does not resemble in any way the electrical activity of the vagotomised stomach described by Kelly and Code (1969).

Reproducibility

The type of electrical activity described is seen in about 70% of preparations. There are obviously different patterns found when there has been some technical error in setting up the experiment, but in 30% variations are seen for which there is, at the present time, no explanation; included in this group are those preparations in which the physical and biochemical monitoring of the perfusion reveals no abnormality. The variations encountered may be listed as follows:

1. Abnormally low frequency of the gastric slow wave often associated with a normal duodenal pattern.
2. Failure of aboral propagation of the slow wave.
3. Abnormal conduction patterns.
4. A normal slow wave, with complete absence of spike potentials.
5. Abnormally fast antral slow wave (antral tachygastria).

These preparations which do not exhibit what we have described as the normal pattern of electrical activity none the less form an interesting group, and they may well shed further light on the complex problem of the integration of gastro-intestinal motor activity. If the other parameters of perfusion data are within the acceptable limits they should be retained and studied as a separate group.

Mechanical Activity

Methods

Intraluminal pressure changes in the antrum and duodenum may be recorded using water filled non-perfused open tipped tubes 1 mm in diameter. These will reflect the mechanical activity of the wall in a narrow lumen viscus, but to record this from the body and fundus of the stomach the use of fluid filled balloons is to be preferred.

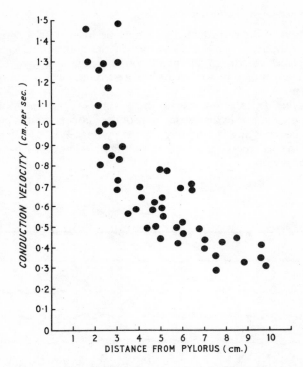

Fig. 46 The inter electrode propagation velocity of the pacesetter potential is shown here and related to a number of different sites on the stomach. Note the gradual increase in velocity in the body and proximal antrum and the much more pronounced increase as the potential approaches the pylorus.

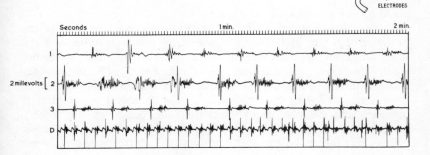

Fig. 47 Electrode D shows the Duodenal pacesetter potential and spike activity. In this preparation the frequency was 17/minute and no relationship between gastric and duodenal slow wave or spike activity can be seen.

Introduction of the recording device may be by way of a spool tied into the oesophagus, or the distal part of the duodenum. The units may be placed *in situ*, or the pull-through technique employed with particular advantage in studies on the gastro-duodenal junction and oesophagus.

By placing an infusion tube in the gastro-oesophageal sphincter, and a collecting tube in the second part of the duodenum, it is possible to study the emptying of fluid through the pylorus. We have employed the same ink-jet recording system in motility studies as we have used for electrical work.

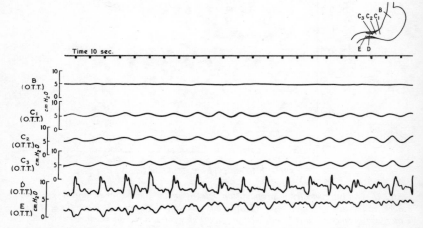

Fig. 48 A recording demonstrating the differing rates of antral (C 1–3) and duodenal (E) contraction waves. Note the high pressure waves seen in the pylorus (D) which occur in relation to the second half of the antral contractions.

Motility of the Unstimulated Preparation

The resting intragastric pressure relative to atmospheric is in the order of 2–4 cm of water as measured by open tip tube, and the intra-duodenal pressure a centimetre or two less. Regular 5/min contractions are recorded from the antrum and 17–19/min contractions from the duodenum (Figure 48). In addition a steep rise in pressure, timed with the second half of each antral contraction is found, using the pull-through technique, to occur only in a very narrow zone between 0·8 and 1·2 cm in length (Figure 49). Either side of this region, typical antral or duodenal contractions are always recorded. Using the pull-through technique we find also that the typical pyloric contractions are superimposed upon a zone of raised pressure 3–4 cm above intragastric pressure, and between 0·8 to 1·2 cm in length. These observations on the gastro-duodenal junction in the isolated preparation are similar to those of Brink *et al* (1965) in the intact animal.

The fact that the preparation exhibits continuous spontaneous motility is advantageous not only for a study of the mechanisms which may inhibit it, but also for investigation into the control of gastro-duodenal motility, and the regulation of gastric emptying.

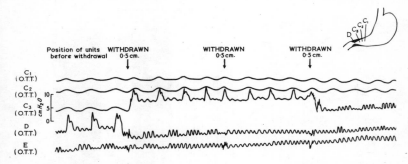

Fig. 49 A pressure profile of the gastro-duodenal junction. Note that the large pyloric contractions are superimposed on the zone of elevated pressure.

Acid Secretion

It has been well demonstrated by Lim *et al* (1927), Dristas and Kowalewski (1966) and Way and Hawley (1970), that the isolated stomach preparation, perfused by cross-circulation with another animal will secrete acid in response to histamine. Salmon and Assimocopoulos (1964) using an isolated circuit, but the lung of the donor animal as the method of oxygenation, obtained acid secretion in response to histamine in only 30% of their preparations. They suggested that prolonged anoxia, and the use of homologous donor blood accounted for some of the failures. Moody *et al* (1962) constructed wedge preparations of gastric fundus and obtained brisk acid secretion in response to histamine. However, he found, as did Way and Hawley, that if the perfusion of the preparation was transferred to an isolated pump-oxygenator circuit, then the acid response disappeared quite quickly despite continued infusion of histamine.

It has been our experience that the isolated perfused stomach preparation does not secrete acid in response to an infusion of histamine, and our observations would further suggest that this is a complete block to any secretory response, as we have never seen an increase either in the volume of gastric secretion or in its hydrogen ion content.

Cross-circulation studies with the circuit shown in Figure 40 p. 142, in which the same system of pump and tubing is used as in the truly isolated studies, have clearly shown that this preparation is capable of a sustained acid response to an intra-arterial infusion of histamine at a dose of 20 micrograms/min (Figure 50).

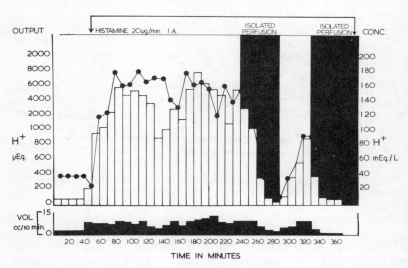

Fig. 50 Note the acid secretory response to histamine in the cross perfused stomach which is abolished by switching to isolated perfusion.

The nature of this block to secretion is at the present time undetermined. It is a complete block, not only to histamine and a number of histamine derivatives, but to gastrin and pentagastrin as well. We have so far identified no physical or biochemical difference between the secreting and non-secreting preparations; the parameters of electrical activity and motility appear the same in both situations; as do measurements of the transmucosal potential difference. Using a Xenon[133] washout technique we have shown that mucosal perfusion with blood is the same whether the stomach is secreting or not, and it would appear therefore that it is not a failure of the blood supply to the parietal cell that is the cause of its inability to secrete.

It is of further interest that these observations have recently been confirmed by Kowalewski and Scharf (1971) using a similar preparation.

We have no other evidence that the preparation suffers by virtue of its isolation and we believe it still to be of value for physiologic studies despite this remarkable defect in its performance.

Assessment of the Gastro-oesophageal Junction

Introduction
Much has been written in the past twenty years about the factors involved in the prevention of oesophageal reflux. There is no doubt that there are many mechanisms involved and that they all combine to protect the lower oesophagus from gastric contents. Many of these are anatomical, e.g. the oesophago-gastric angle, the diaphragmatic crura and the gastric mucosal rosette, but probably the most important single factor is the physiological gastro-oesophageal sphincter (Ingram *et al*, 1959; Mann *et al*, 1964 (i); Vandertoll *et al*, 1966). Earlier work assessed the relative importance of each of the mechanisms (Vantrappen *et al*, 1960; Mann *et al*, 1964 (ii)). In addition, attention was directed to establishing the basic physiology of the gastro-oesophageal sphincter. Most of this work has been performed on either humans (Fyke *et al*, 1956) or on isolated sphincteric muscle strips (Christensen, 1970). The development of an isolated canine gastro-oesophageal sphincter preparation is an attempt to bridge the gap between the above two experimental methods. If the isolated preparation can be shown to behave in a similar fashion to that seen in intact animals then it is feasible to use it as a basis for a further study on the factors affecting the physiological sphincter.

This preparation has therefore been assessed in terms relating to accepted functions of the gastro-oesophageal sphincter area of the human and the intact dog. These are:

1. Pressure measurements
2. Responses to oesophageal balloon distension
3. Mucosal potential difference measurements
4. Sphincteric electrical activity

Pressure Measurements
Intraluminal pressures were recorded as detecting units were withdrawn at 0·5 cm intervals from the fundus into the body of the oesophagus. The unit consisted either of a non-infused water-filled side open-tipped tube or of a small balloon 0·5 cm in diameter. The transducers were adjusted to lie at the same level as the preparation. Figure 51 is an example of such a pull-through using a balloon unit.

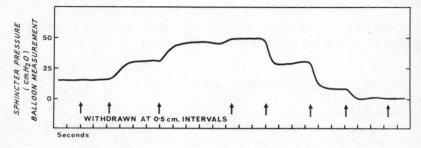

Fig. 51 A pressure profile of the gastro-oesophageal sphincter. A balloon manometer has been withdrawn at 0·5 cm intervals from the fundus of the stomach into the body of the oesophagus.

There are, of course, no respiratory waves and points of respiratory reversal to mark the position of the diaphragmatic hiatus. Data taken from 250 open-tip pull-through studies show that the mean sphincteric pressure was $15·0 \pm 8·5$ cm water above atmospheric pressure. These values are similar to those in the intact dog (Schlegel and Code, 1958). The lengths of the zone of elevated pressure as measured by open-tip recordings were $2·2 \pm 0·7$ cm. This is also in agreement with the work quoted above.

It will be noted from the size of the standard deviation that there can be a great difference in the sphincter pressures from one preparation to the next. However, Figure 52 demonstrates that for

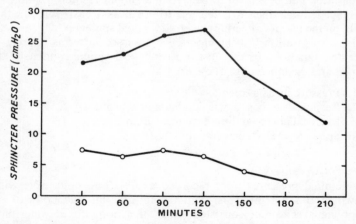

Fig. 52 Two examples of the mean gastro-oesophageal sphincteric pressures over the first three hours of perfusion. Note the steady pressure for the first two hours which is followed by a gradual decline in pressure.

any one study, the sphincteric pressure remains constant for the first two hours and then begins to fall off. All pressure studies should therefore be performed during this initial period.

Responses to Oesophageal Balloon Distension
It has been demonstrated in humans by Creamer and Schlegel (1957) that oesophageal balloon distension will produce relaxation of the gastro-oesophageal sphincter but no distal oesophageal peristaltic waves. If 50 cc of water are used as a distending force then both a peristaltic wave and sphincteric relaxation are seen. Figure 53 shows the response of the isolated gastro-oesophageal sphincter to balloon distension of the body of the oesophagus.

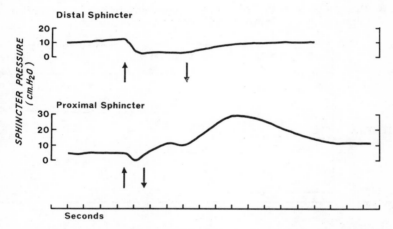

Fig. 53 *The responses of the gastro-oesophageal sphincter to oesophageal balloon distension. Note the relaxation in the distal sphincter, and the relaxation followed by a contraction in the proximal part of the sphincter.*

The two halves of the sphincter respond differently. The distal part relaxes and then returns to its previous pressure, whereas the proximal sphincter relaxes initially but is then followed by a contraction. These responses are identical to the sphincteric deglutitive responses seen in intact dogs and humans (Kelley Jr *et al,* 1960). No peristaltic waves have been recorded from the body of the oesophagus.

Mucosal Potential Difference Measurements
Potential difference measurements were made at the same time as the pressure recordings using a technique developed by Helm *et al,* (1965). It

has been shown in humans (Helm *et al*, 1965) and in dogs (Greenwood *et al*, 1965) that the site of maximal change in the transmucosal potential difference corresponded to the gastro-oesophageal mucosal junction, and that on withdrawing the exploring electrode from the fundus of the stomach into the body of the oesophagus there is a reversal of the potential difference from negative to positive.

An open-tip tube was filled with saturated potassium chloride in Agar gel and was attached to a separate pressure recording line. The potential difference line was connected to a beaker filled with saturated potassium chloride. A similar line, used as the reference electrode, was placed on the serosa of the stomach and its other end connected to another beaker of saturated potassium chloride. Into each beaker was placed a mercury/mercuric chloride electrode and each was connected to a potentiometer. In addition, the potential difference was recorded simultaneously on a Mingograf 81 recording apparatus.

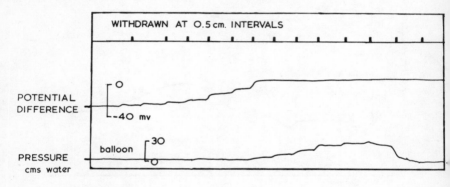

Fig. 54 A simultaneous pressure and potential difference profile of the gastro-oesophageal sphincter. Note the gradual change of polarity between the stomach and the oesophagus which lies within the zone of elevated pressure.

Figure 54 shows a simultaneous recording of the pressure and potential difference change as the detecting units were pulled through the gastro-oesophageal junction. The potential difference in the stomach was –30 millivolts, and in the oesophagus it was +5 millivolts. There is a zone of transition which falls within the zone of elevated pressure. This confirms that in the isolated preparation the gastro-oesophageal mucosal junction lies within the sphincter area and agrees with the work of the above authors on the human and the intact dog.

Electrical Activity

Technique

Two electrode sites are used. Both are on the gastro-oesophageal sphincter; one above the phreno-oesophageal membrane and the other below it (Figure 55). It has been found to be easier to attach the electrodes before the preparation is removed from the donor animal. This is most suitably done after the oesophagus has been freed from the posterior chest wall.

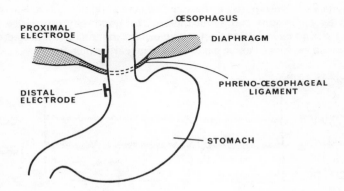

Fig. 55 A diagram showing the sites of the two electrodes on the gastro-oesophageal sphincter. One is above and the other below the diaphragm.

Both electrodes are attached in the transverse axis of the oeso-phagus. The sphincteric zone is coloured white and its upper limit is easily distinguished from the red striated muscle of the body of the oesophagus. The proximal electrode is attached just above the diaphragm, and this is a simple procedure. Implantation of the distal electrode is more difficult. The cut edge of the lesser omentum is lifted clear of the intra-abdominal segment of the oesophagus. It is usual to find a clear area on the sphincteric zone at a point where the lesser curve of the stomach joins the oesophagus. The many small vessels in this area must be avoided as haemorrhage in this confined space will interfere with the electrical recording.

Silver/silver chloride bipolar electrodes are used. Their tips are set 5 mm apart and are 5 mm long. The electrical activity is recorded on an eight-channel recording apparatus (Mingograf 81). Spike activity is recorded at a time constant of 0·03 seconds and filtered at 15 Hertz.

Recordings
Two groups of workers (Hellemans and Vantrappen, 1967, Hellemans *et al,* 1968, Arimori *et al,* 1970) have previously studied the electrical activity from the intact canine gastro-oesophageal sphincter. These workers agree that the electrical activity recorded from the infra- and supra-diaphragmatic parts of the sphincter differ. Both groups recognise sphincteric action potentials occurring in the proximal part of the sphincter which are related to sphincteric contraction. They also agree that such action potentials are not seen in the infra-diaphragmatic portion. Arimori *et al* (1970) recorded a continuous phasic electrical activity from both parts of the sphincter. Such phasic activity was not seen by Hellemans and Vantrappen (1967) and they concluded that there was a marked discordance between the manometric and electrical observations in the canine gastro-oesophageal sphincter.

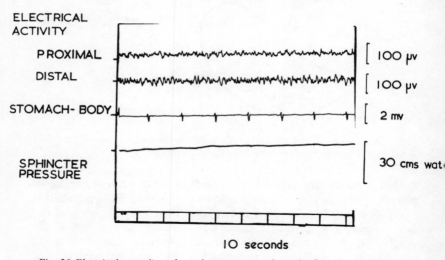

Fig. 56 Electrical recordings from the gastro-oesophageal sphincter in a preparation where the sphincteric pressure remains constant. Note the irregular 50 micro volt activity recorded from above and below the diaphragm.

In the isolated preparation phasic electrical activity has been recorded from both parts of the sphincter. If sphincteric pressures were continually monitored and related to the electrical recordings, two basic electrical patterns could be distinguished. In those preparations where the resting sphincteric pressure, as measured by an indwelling balloon manometer, was constant, an irregular 50-microvolt wave pattern was recorded from both electrical sites (Figure 56).

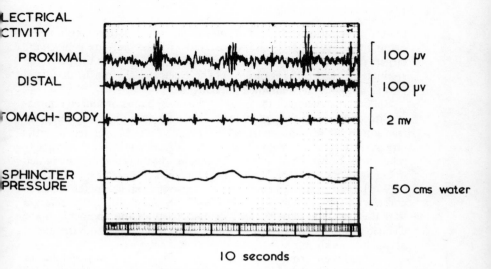

Fig. 57 *Electrical recordings from the gastro-oesophageal sphincter in a preparation where the sphincter was undergoing phasic contractions. Note the action potentials associated with the rise in sphincteric pressure.*

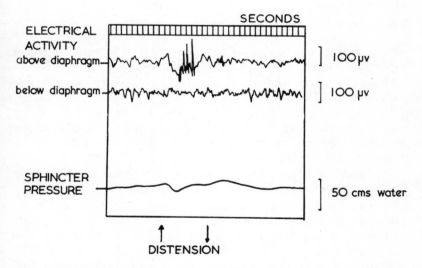

Fig. 58 *Electrical and manometric responses to oesophageal balloon distension. Note action potentials in the proximal part of the sphincter which coincides with sphincteric contraction. The electrical activity in the distal part of the sphincter is diminished and corresponds to the sphincteric relaxation.*

Other preparations showed a phasic pressure pattern with peaks occurring every 30 seconds. Associated with the pressure peaks were larger, faster action potentials which were only seen in the proximal sphincteric electrode (Figure 57). The electrical rhythm in the distal part of the sphincter remained unchanged.

Balloon distension of the body of the oesophagus produced characteristic changes in the sphincteric electrical activity. The after contraction in the proximal part of the sphincter was associated with the larger, faster action potentials. In the distal sphincter where only relaxation occurs, the phasic electrical rhythm usually remained unchanged but occasionally it was diminished (Figure 58).

Work on the isolated canine gastro-oesophageal sphincter seems to agree with that of Arimori *et al* (1970) on intact dogs. It is thought that the base-line activity seen in both parts of the sphincter is the electrical equivalent of the resting sphincteric tone and the faster action potentials represent sphincteric contraction.

It would seem from these studies that the isolated perfused canine gastro-oesophageal sphincter exhibits the main physiological properties usually seen in the intact lower oesophageal sphincter. The preparation is offered as an additional experimental method for studying the gastro-oesophageal junction.

References

Allen, G.L., Poole, E.W. and Code, C.F. (1964) Relationship between electrical activities of antrum and duodenum *Am. J. Physiol.* **207,** 906.

Alvarez, W.C. and Mahoney, L.J. (1922) Action currents in stomach and intestine. *Am. J. Physiol.* **58,** 476.

Arimori, M., Code, C.F., Schlegel, J.F. and Sturm, R.E. (1970) Electrical activity of the canine oesophagus and gastro-oesophageal sphincter: its relation to intra-luminal pressure and movement of material. *Amer. J. Dig. Dis.* **15,** 191.

Brink, B.M., Schlegel, J.F. and Code, C.F. (1965) The pressure profile of the gastro-duodenal junctional zone in dogs. *Gut* **6,** 163.

Christensen, J. (1970) Pharmacologic identification of the lower oesophageal sphincter. *J. Clin. Invest.* **49,** 681.

Creamer, B. and Schlegel, J. (1957) Motor responses of the oesophagus to distension. *J. Appl. Physiol.* **10,** 498.

Daniel, E.E. and Chapman, K.M. (1963) The electrical activity of the gastrointestinal tract as an indication of mechanical activity. *Amer. J. Dig. Dis.* **8,** 54.

Dritsas, K.G. Bondar, G.F. and Kowalewski, K. (1966) Secretory response to sustained histamine stimulation of the isolated canine stomach. *Brit. J. Surg.* **53,** 798.

Dritsas, K.G. and Kowalewski, K. (1966) Perfusion of the isolated stomach. *Brit. J. Surg.* **53,** 732.

Fyke, F.E. Jr., Code, C.F. and Schlegel, J.F. (1956) The gastro-oesophageal sphincter in healthy human beings. *Gastroenterologie* (Basal), **86,** 135.

Green, W.E.R. and Hardcastle, J.D. (1970) A technique of perfusion of the isolated canine stomach. *J. Physiol.* **208,** 9 P.

Green, W.E.R., Hardcastle, J.D. and Ritchie, H.D. (1970) The myoelectrical activity of the isolated perfused canine stomach. *Brit. J. Surg.* **57,** 858.

Green, W.E.R. and Hardcastle, J.D. (1970) The effect of drugs on the junctional zone of the isolated perfused stomach and duodenum. 4th World Congress of Gastroenterology. Copenhagen 083 Abstracts.

Greenwood, R.K., Schlegel, J.F., Helm, W.J. and Code, C.F. (1965) Pressure and potential difference characteristics of surgically-created hiatal hernia. *Gastroenterology* **48,** 602.

Hellemans, J. and Vantrappen, G. (1967) Electromyographic studies on canine oesophageal motility. *Amer. J. Dig. Dis.* **12,** 1240.

Hellemans, J., Vantrappen, G., Valembois, P., Janssens, J. and Van Den Brouck, J. (1968) Electrical activity of striated and smooth muscle of the oesophagus. *Amer. J. Dig. Dis.* **13,** 320.

Helm, W.J., Schlegel, J.F., Code, C.F. and Summerskill, W.H.J. (1965) Identification of the gastro-oesophageal mucosal junction by trans-mucosal potential in healthy subjects and patients with hiatus hernia. *Gastroenterology,* **48,** 25.

Hermon-Taylor, J. and Code, C.F. (1971) Localisation of the duodenal pacemaker and its role in the organisation of duodenal myoelectric activity. *Gut* **12,** 40.

Ingram, P.R., Respess, J.C. and Muller, W.H. Jr. (1959) The role of the intrinsic sphincter mechanism in the prevention of reflux oeso-phagitis. *Surg. Gynec. Obstet.* **109,** 659.

Kelley, M.L. Jr., Wilbur, D.L. III, Schlegel, J.F. and Code, C.F. (1960) Deglutition responses in the gastro-oesophageal sphincter of healthy human beings. *J. Appl. Physiol.* **15,** 483.

Kelly, K.A., Code, C.F. and Elveback, L.R. (1969) Patterns of canine gastric electrical activity. *Amer. J. Physiol.* **217,** 461.

Kelly, K.A. and Code, C.F. (1969) The effect of transthoracic vagotomy on canine gastric electrical activity. *Gastroenterology* **57**, 51.

Kowalewski, K. and Scharf, R. (1971) Secretion of hydrochloric acid by *ex vivo* isolated canine stomach. *Scand. J. Gastroent.* **6,** 675.

Lim, Robert Kmo-Seng, Loo, Chih-Te and Liu, An-Ch'ang. (1927) Observations on the secretion of the transplanted stomach. *Chinese J. Physiol.* **1,** 56.

Lim, R.K.S., Necheles, M. and Hou, H.C. (1927) The influence of meals on the acutely denervated (vivi-perfused) stomach. *Chinese J. Physiol.* **1,** 263.

Lim, R.K.S., Necheles, M. and Ni, T.G. (1927) The vasomotor reactions of the (vivi-perfused) stomach. *Chinese J. Physiol.* **1,** 381.

Mann, C.V., Ellis, F.H. Jr., Schlegel, J.F. and Code, C.F. (1964) Abdominal displacement of the canine gastro-oesophageal sphincter. *Surg. Gynec. Obstet.* **118,** 1009.

Mann, C.V., Greenwood, R.K. and Ellis, F.H. Jr. (1964) The oesophago-gastric junction. *Surg. Gynec. Obstet.* **118,** 853.

Miller, R.A. and Benfey, B.G. (1958) The fluorimetric estimation of adrenaline and noradrenaline during haemorrhagic hypotension. *Brit. J. Anaesth.* **30,** 158.

Moody, F.G., Gilder, M. and Beal, J.M. (1962) Perfusion secretory studies of the isolated canine stomach. *Surg. Forum* **13,** 282.

Salmon, P.A. and Assimacopoulos, C.A. (1964) Perfusion of the isolated canine stomach. A preliminary report. *J. Surg. Res.* **4,** 339.

Schlegel, J.F. and Code, C.F. (1958) Pressure characteristics of the oesophagus and its sphincters in dogs. *Amer. J. Physiol.* **193,** 9.

Vandertoll, D.J., Ellis, F.H. Jr., Schlegel, J.F. and Code, C.F. (1966) An experimental study of the role of the gastric and oesophageal muscle in gastro-oesophageal competence. *Surg. Gynec. Obstet.* **122,** 579.

Vantrappen, G., Clinton Texter, E. Jr., Barboka, C.J. and Vandenbrouck, E. (1960) The closing mechanism at the gastro-oesophageal junction. *Amer. J. Med.* **28,** 564.

Way, L.W. and Hawley, P.R. (1969) Isolated perfusion of the canine stomach. *Surg. Gynec. Obstet.* **129,** 1005.

Weber, J. Jr. and Kohatsu, S. (1970) Pacemaker localization and electrical conduction pattern in the canine stomach. *Gastroenterology,* **59,** 717.

CHAPTER TEN

Duodenum and Pancreas

The Isolated Perfused Canine Pancreas

Introduction

It should be remembered that the preparation of an isolated perfused pancreas is not an end in itself; it establishes the pancreas in circumstances in which it is easily studied. The initial objective of the research worker should therefore be to achieve the degree of expertise necessary to set up the preparation as quickly and simply as possible, and to concentrate his efforts on subsequent experiments. The investigator should bear in mind that although the operation is not being performed on a patient this does not mean that the standard of surgery may in any way be reduced. There must be a good light, a good assistant and good instruments, and since the investigator is unlikely to be assisted by a nurse, he must himself ensure that the operative area and instruments are kept clean. The only concession made is that sterile procedure can be omitted since in this instance the animal does not survive.

Isolated perfusion of the canine pancreas was described by Babkin and Starling in 1926 and refined and developed by Nardi and his colleagues in 1965. This is not, therefore, the first description of the preparation, but is a method which ensures that the whole pancreas is consistently perfused using relatively simple apparatus (Hermon-Taylor, 1968). The following detailed account is intended to serve as a guide to those workers who may be interested in this field.

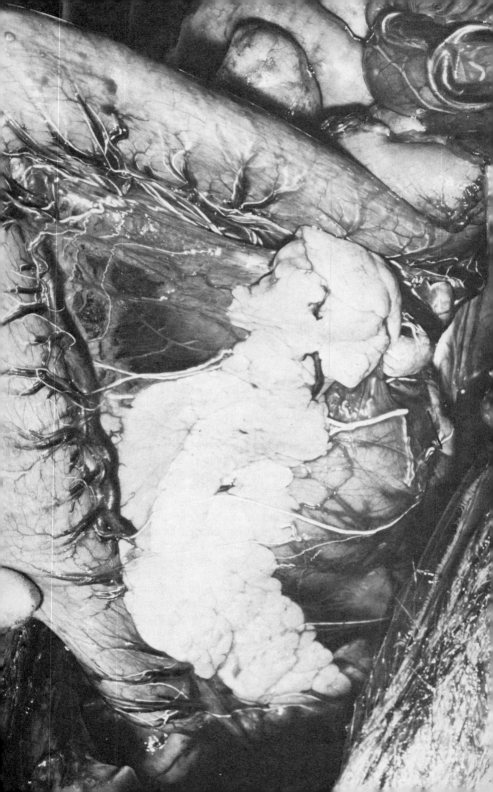

Anatomy

The pancreas of a dog is a delicate, finely lobulated yellowish structure weighing 40 to 60 g. As in man the head is closely related to the concavity of the duodenal loop; the body and tail of the gland extends to the left, crossing the coeliac axis and lying along the splenic vessels. The tail ends some distance from the hilum of the spleen. The uncinate process arises from the caudal aspect of the head of the pancreas and extends to the left away from the duodenum. The duodenum itself does not occupy the retro-peritoneal position it does in man, but is attached to a well-developed mesentery in which part of the pancreas lies. The pancreas and duodenal loop can, therefore, be lifted up out of the abdomen (Figure 59). The fourth part of the duodenum is connected to the posterior abdominal wall by a tri-angular leaf of peritoneum, which has a lower crescentic free margin and apex at the root of the superior mesenteric artery. The thin upper border of the body and tail of the pancreas is attached throughout its length to a mesentery which is continuous with the right-hand edge of the greater omentum.

Arterial Supply

The resting blood flow of the canine pancreas has been estimated to be 0·6 ml per gramme per minute (Delaney and Custer, 1965) and is derived from the coeliac and superior mesenteric arterial systems (Figure 60). One or two short branches from the splenic artery enter the tail of the pancreas near its tip; a larger artery enters the body of the pancreas from the splenic, arising near its origin from the coeliac. Occasionally this vessel comes from the first few millimetres of the left gastric artery.

The hepatic artery is easily recognised running up towards the liver surrounded by a conspicuous plexus of nerves. Near the hilum it gives off a large branch, the superior pancreatico-duodenal which curves downwards and enters the junction of the proximal duodenum and pancreas. Just before entering the pancreas this vessel gives a branch to the first part of the duodenum. In the gland a second branch runs to the left in the body of the pancreas to anastomose with the splenic branches (Figure 61). Thereafter the superior pancreatico-duodenal artery continues downwards in the head of the gland and ends by anastomosing with the terminal branch of the inferior pancreatico-duodenal. This junction is small.

The inferior pancreatico-duodenal artery supplies the uncinate process and arises from the right hand side of the superior mesenteric artery about 3 cm from its origin on the aorta. At first it runs

59 Photograph from the right side of the animal showing duodenum held up out
he abdomen. The duodenal mesentery contains the head and uncinate processes of
pancreas.

downwards closely related to other vessels in the root of the mesentery, but it then passes to the right, gives several branches to the duodenum and enters the uncinate process. It ends by anastomosing with the superior vessel. Under normal circumstances the inferior pancreatico-duodenal artery is the only contribution to pancreatic blood supply made from the superior mesenteric, but on occasions branches from the splenic artery may be absent, and the body of the gland is supplied by a large branch arising directly from the trunk of

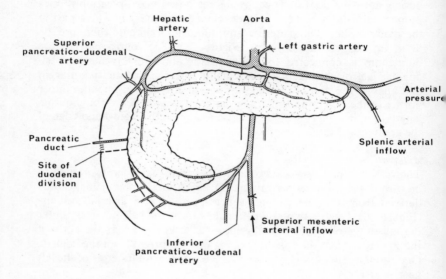

Fig. 60 Normal arterial supply of the canine pancreas from the coeliac and superior mesenteric arterial systems.

the superior mesenteric. Such anomalies of the arterial supply and small size of arterial anastomoses underline the importance of perfusing both coeliac and superior mesenteric systems if consistently viable preparations are to be obtained.

Venous Drainage

The smaller veins run alongside the arteries. The inferior pancreatico-duodenal vein drains into the superior mesenteric which receives the splenic vein and runs up behind the neck of the pancreas and duodenum (Figure 62). Occasionally the inferior pancreatico-duodenal vein is small or absent in which case blood from the

Fig. 61 Arteriogram of the isolated perfused pancreas and short attached portion duodenum. The coeliac and superior mesenteric arterial cannulas are seen to the right of illustration. The cannula in the pancreatic duct opacifies on the left.

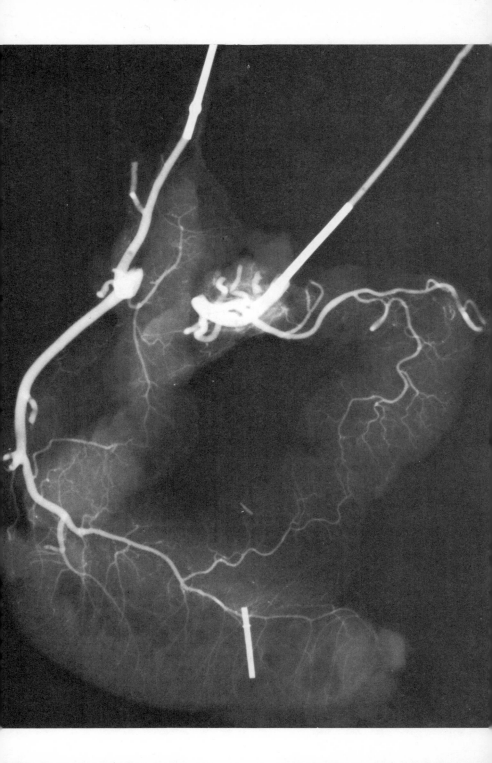

uncinate process drains via the superior pancreatico-duodenal. This vessel runs upwards in the posterior groove between the pancreas and duodenum and enters the right side of the portal vein behind the upper border of the first part of the duodenum. From this point the definitive portal vein is wide, but short, and only runs for 1 to 2 cm before it divides to enter the liver.

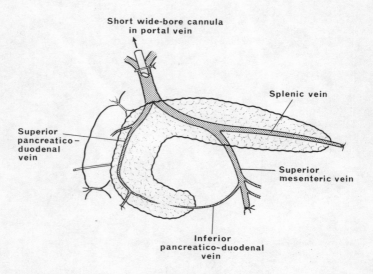

Fig. 62 Diagram of venous drainage of the canine pancreas showing portal venous cannula in position.

Duct System

The main pancreatic duct in the dog does not enter the duodenum at the biliary ampulla as in man, but about 2 cm distal to it. On opening the duodenum the pancreatic ampulla is seen as a slightly raised, pale area 2 to 3 mm in diameter with the lumen of the pancreatic duct in its centre (Figure 63). It lies just on the anterior side of the medial margin of the duodenum about 5 cm distal to the pylorus. It possesses a well marked sphincter which is felt as the orifice is cannulated.

The main duct draining the body and tail of the pancreas runs in the centre of that part of the gland and turns downwards in the head of the pancreas to enter the duodenum. Just before it passes through the duodenal wall it receives the duct of the uncinate process (Figure

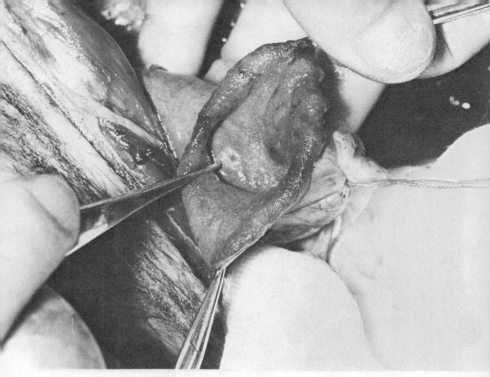

Fig. 63 The main pancreatic duct is seen on opening the duodenum.

64). The accessory pancreatic duct is very small; when present it runs from the main duct to the duodenum at the biliary ampulla. The volume of the duct system of the pancreas varies from about 0·8 to 1·5 ml. This should be taken into account when interpreting changes in composition of pancreatic secretion following stimuli which have only a small effect on the basal rate of flow.

Apparatus

The perfusion apparatus must clearly be ready before embarking on the operation. The characteristics of various types of equipment have been discussed in Chapter 5. For pancreatic perfusion the circuit is centred upon a Perspex water bath maintained at 38°C and placed on a stand at the end of the operating table (Figures 65 & 66). It is convenient if the height of the table can be adjusted so as to vary the pressure of venous return. A small disc oxygenator is mounted in the top of the bath with the level of the water just below the central bearing which may leak. The oxygenator is driven by a small electric

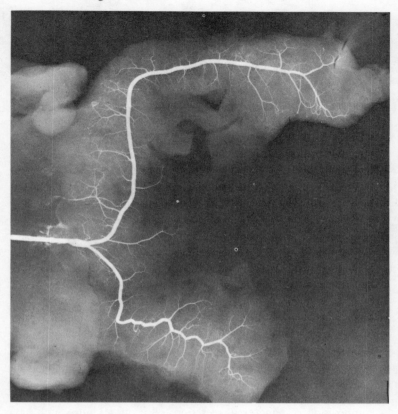

Fig. 64 Radiograph of pancreatic duct system of the dog showing cannula in main pancreatic ampulla. The accessory pancreatic duct is seen as a very small connection with the duodenum proximal to the main opening.

motor geared so that the discs rotate at about 10 rpm. This is sufficient to maintain a continuous film of blood on the discs and an arterial oxygen saturation of 100% at blood flow rate of 15 to 20 ml/min. Frothing does not occur and blood damage is minimised. Alternatively a disposable bubble oxygenator may be used mounted on a burette stand in the water bath. In this case the flow rate of gas to the oxygenating column should be as low as possible so that the bubbles just reach the surface.

The arterial line between the oxygenator and the pump should contain a coil of tubing to act as a heat exchanger and a side tap for

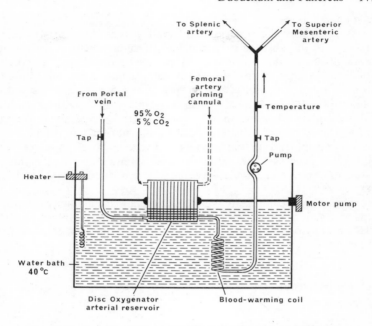

To Splenic artery

To Superior Mesenteric artery

Femoral artery priming cannula

From Portal vein

95% O₂
5% CO₂

Temperature

Tap

Tap

Pump

Heater

Motor pump

Water bath
40 °C

Disc Oxygenator
arterial reservoir

Blood-warming coil

Fig. 65 Diagram of perfusion circuit for isolated pancreatic perfusion.

sampling arterial blood and infusion of test substances. An infusion is thus warmed as it reaches the arterial line. The pump is placed by the side of the water bath and the tubing beyond it contains the temperature probe, and if necessary a flow meter. It ends in a reduction Y junction, the limbs of which later receive tubing from the splenic and superior mesenteric arterial cannulae.

The venous line contains a side tap for sampling blood; it may also be used for discarding the venous return for an interval following the injection of a test substance into the arterial line, to prevent the bolus entering the perfusion circuit. The preparation is contained in a closed Perspex box with appropriate slots in the side to admit tubing. This box is placed close to the water bath and pump, reducing the length of exposed tubing, and preventing wide fluctuations in temperature of the blood as it passes round the circuit. Thus arranged the total volume of the perfusion circuit is about 750 ml. Should more arterial blood from the animal be available it may be stored in a separate bottle in the water bath or a reservoir incorporated in the arterial line. At low flow rates storage of deoxygenated blood in a venous reservoir may lead to stagnation and acidosis and should be avoided.

Cannulae

It is important not to cannulate small vessels directly with plastic tubing. In the absence of a shoulder, if such tubing is tied in tight enough not to slip out it will sometimes be obstructed, and if it is tied in so that obstruction does not occur, some will slip out. Simple tubular cannulae of appropriate size for the arteries and the duct should be made of polished stainless steel with a shoulder above which a ligature may be placed with confidence. In the case of the duct cannula this shoulder should not be more than 2 or 3 mm from the end, or the cannula will tend to block the duct of the uncinate process. The portal venous cannula may be nylon or stainless steel and should have an internal diameter of about 0·5 cm.

The arterial cannulae have the same diameter as the two limbs of the Y junction in the arterial line and should each be attached to 10 to 15 cm of nylon tubing filled with heparinised saline and clamped prior to surgery.

Operative Details

Design

The operation is designed so that at no time in the transference to artificial perfusion is the pancreas deprived of an arterial blood supply. The spleen, stomach and intestine are removed in turn, isolating the pancreatic circulation. The perfusion circuit is primed with oxygenated blood from a femoral artery and connected to cannulae placed retrogradely in the splenic and superior mesenteric arteries, and perfusion started. The origins of the coeliac and superior mesenteric arteries are then ligated on the aorta and the animal bled out rapidly into the circuit. It then remains to exclude the liver, cannulate the portal vein and establish the preparation in its artificial environment.

Operative Procedure

The dog is anaesthetised with Pentobarbitone, placed on an operating table, intubated, and positive pressure ventilation with 100% oxygen is started. A midline abdominal incision is made. It is important to pay attention to haemostasis as blood lost from the wound, especially after heparinisation, will reduce the amount subsequently available to prime the perfusion circuit. Greyhounds do not have a good linea alba and the peritoneal vessels should be diathermied before the peritoneum is opened. It is important to carry

Fig. 66 Photograph of apparatus. Disc oxygenator and water bath are seen to the left of frame and infusion pump on the right.

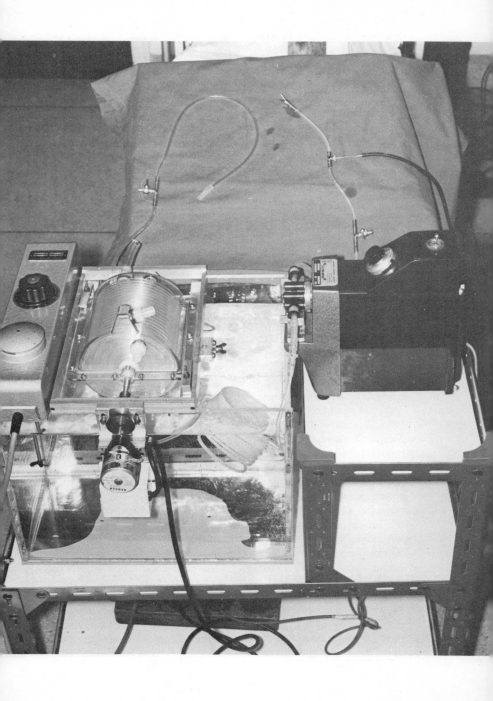

the incision right up to the xiphisternum, avoiding the terminal branch of the internal mammary artery. Once the abdomen is opened a self-retaining retractor is put in place. A useful way of doing this is to have a hook on the abdominal wall tied out to the side of the table. The splanchnic vessels in dogs are not usually obscured by mesenteric fat and are easily seen; it is more precise to ligate them before division, rather than clamp the vessels and then ligate them, as it is less traumatic and helps to avoid haematoma formation after heparinisation. A most useful instrument for the purpose is a fully curved Stille forceps.

Spleen The first manoeuvre is to lift the spleen out of the abdomen, and while the assistant holds it downwards, ligate and divide the gastro-splenic vessels in one or two pedicles. The operator should then gather up the right-hand edge of the omentum which has the body and tail of the pancreas in its extremity. As the manoeuvre is completed this part of the pancreas emerges into view together with two or three small vessels that connect with this mesentery. The assistant supports the greater omentum while these vessels are carefully ligated and the mesentery divided. The remaining part of the greater omentum can then be detached from the greater curvature of the stomach. Peritoneal attachments of the splenic hilum to the posterior abdominal wall should be divided in the plane devoid of blood vessels, and the two main branches of the splenic artery tied individually, the ligatures being left long to facilitate subsequent retrieval and cannulation. The spleen is removed.

Stomach The next step is to find the pylorus and cut its suspensory ligament, allowing it to be drawn down a little further. The right gastro-epiploic vessels should be divided between ligatures below the pylorus; the duodenum and gastric antrum are tied firmly with thread either side of the pylorus which is divided. The assistant now lifts the stomach and exposes the left gastric artery and vein arising from the coeliac or occasionally from the splenic (Figure 67). These vessels lie in the free margin of a crescentic fold of connective tissue between the stomach and the right crus of the diaphragm. This fold contains the branches of the posterior vagus passing to the coeliac plexus and frequently a small branch of the coeliac artery which must be secured. The left gastric artery and vein are ligated together and divided. When the artery to the body of the pancreas comes off the left gastric rather than the splenic, it must be carefully preserved. The stomach does not need to be removed and may be pushed back under the left costal margin.

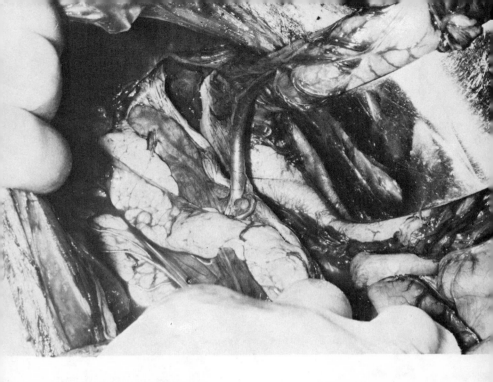

Fig. 67 The left gastric vein with artery behind is seen in the free border of the crescentic fold referred to in the text. The stomach has been retracted. The artery to the body of the pancreas arises near the root of the left gastric artery and curves round to enter this part of the gland.

Small Intestine The assistant should find and hold up the caecum, identified by its somewhat greyer appearance. When this is done, the inferior pancreatico-duodenal vessels come into view, arising out of the root of the mesentery and entering the uncinate process of the pancreas. Preservation of these vessels and retrograde cannulation of the superior mesenteric artery is the most difficult manoeuvre of the operation.

The inferior vessels lie in the mesentery of the duodenum which is in part adherent to the rest of the mesentery of the small intestine. These mesenteries must be separated in the avascular plane between them using fine scissors and non-toothed forceps (Figure 68). When this manoeuvre is completed there is sufficient room to cannulate the superior mesenteric artery retrogradely, distal to the origin of the inferior pancreatico-duodenal. The operator shifts his position so that his part of the superior mesenteric artery is grasped between finger and thumb of the left hand. The right hand is used gently to display the vessel as it lies close against the superior mesenteric vein. Damage

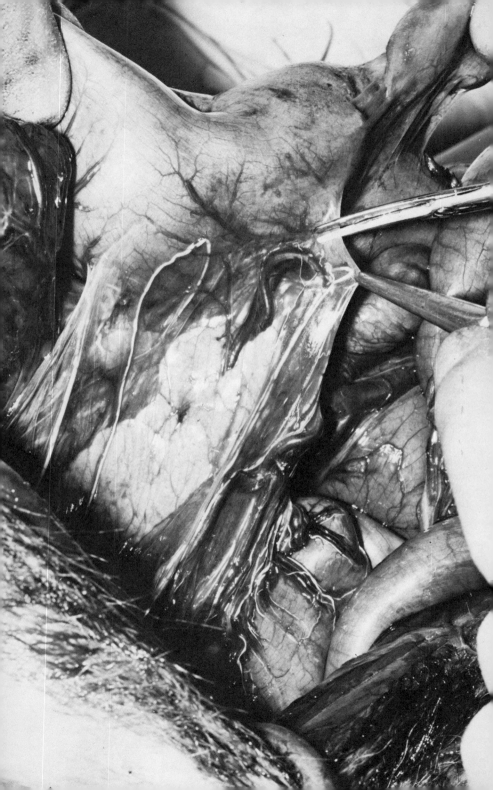

to the small friable vessels which may run with the artery must be avoided, or the main vessel will become obscured by bleeding and the preparation will be ruined by subsequent haematoma formation. With a little practice this is quite easy. A thread ligature is negotiated round the artery using curved forceps, tied by the assistant, and held firmly downwards to put the artery on tension. Another ligature is passed round the vessel but not tied. The operator occludes the root of the mesentery by pinching with the left hand, and cannulates the superior mesenteric artery through a transverse incision. The assistant ties the cannula in place with the proximal ligature. The second ligature should be put round the cannula before the artery is divided beyond it.

The colonic vessels should now be ligated separately and the rest of the root of the mesentery divided between a double ligature. The duodenum is held up and its membranous attachments to the poster-ior abdominal wall divided right down to the root of the superior mesenteric artery. As always in this operation it is helpful to carry out such manoeuvres with light shining through the peritoneal fold so that the course of the scissors may be guided between small vessels. Attention to these details will ensure that blood loss from the heparinised preparation will be negligible. The inferior pancreatico-duodenal artery and vein give a branch to the uncinate process and proceed to the side of the duodenum forming an arcade which re-enters the head of the pancreas in the angle between it and the duodenum (Figure 60). The vessels can usually be ligated beyond the branch to the uncinate process, but on occasions the inferior pan-creatico-duodenal vein may be deficient, and this arcade must be preserved to ensure adequate venous drainage of the uncinate process. A few fine ligatures on the short branches of the arcade will accomplish this without wasting much time. The small intestine is divided just distal to the head of the pancreas. The rectum and the inferior mesenteric artery are now in turn ligated and divided and the intestine removed.

Cannulation of Pancreatic Duct The short duodenal remnant is held up by the assistant using an artery forcep on the distal ligature. The main pancreatic duct will be found at a point about 1 cm proximal to the place where the head of the pancreas leaves its intimate relation with the duodenum to become the uncinate process. Using cutting diathermy a longitudinal incision is made in the ante-mesenteric border centred on this point. The luminal contents are gently mopped out and the orifice of the pancreatic duct identified. It is unwise to make a preliminary exploration of the duct with a probe as it bleeds very easily. It is better to put the cannula straight in and tie it in place

$8 Photograph from the right side of the animal showing coecum held up by the assistant.
ation of the duodenal mesentery containing the inferior pancreaticoèduodenal vessels is
ing in the avascular plain.

with a silk stitch round the ampulla; the cannula should then be gently withdrawn until its shoulder is felt to come up against this ligature. The duct of the uncinate process will then be clear. The duodenotomy is now sutured to prevent bleeding, the cannula being allowed to emerge from between the stitches.

Splenic Arterial Cannulation and Perfusion The stump of the splenic artery is sought and the second arterial cannula is placed in its main branch; the arterial pressure cannula is tied in one of the secondary branches. The femoral vessels are quickly exposed in the right groin and 5 to 10,000 units of heparin injected into the vein. The artery is cannulated and about 200 ml of blood taken into the oxygenator. The arterial side of the circuit is primed and the Y junction connected to the tubing leading to the two arterial cannulae, care being taken to see that air-bubbles are excluded. The clamps are removed and perfusion begun at a low flow rate of 10 to 15 ml/min, since at this stage it is important that the gland should not be overperfused. The clamp is removed from the femoral arterial cannula, and the animal rapidly bled; at the same time the root of the superior mesenteric and coeliac arteries are ligated on the aorta. The ligatures should be as close as possible to the aorta to avoid an anomalous vessel to the body of the pancreas from the superior mesenteric and the hepatic artery which may be inadvertently ligated, as the main trunk of the coeliac is usually not more than 1 cm long. It is not necessary at this stage to divide the origins of these vessels as this can be done at the end of the operation when the circulation of the animal has ceased.

Portal Venous Cannulation A median sternotomy is now made as rapidly as possible. The right diaphragm is divided and an incision extending through the costal margin is made in a right lower intercostal space. By this time the animal will have been bled into the perfusion apparatus. The liver may be reflected into the right pleural cavity, widely exposing the structures at its hilum. A single ligature is placed above the origin of the superior pancreatico-duodenal artery to include the hepatic artery and bile duct. The duodenum is reflected to the left and held by the assistant while the surgeon ligates a duct on the back of the portal vein. A ligature is passed round the portal vein, which is now the only structure attaching the preparation to the liver, and a wide-bore cannula tied into it. Once again this manoeuvre is facilitated by holding the portal vein between the finger and thumb of the left hand. The portal vein above the cannula is detached from the liver. It is important to ensure that venous congestion does not occur and the height of the operating table above the perfusion circuit should be adjusted. It is also important that the portal vein should be cannulated as high up as possible, otherwise the cannula may obstruct the confluence of the superior pancreatico-duodenal and portal veins. The isolated perfused pancreas and short attached portion of duodenum is lifted out and placed in the perfusion chamber. With practice the operation should be completed in one hour.

Establishment of Steady State Conditions

Once the preparation has been placed in the perfusion chamber, at least 30 minutes should be allowed to elapse before any studies are carried out, since the organ takes some time to achieve steady state conditions in its artificial environment.

The arterial and venous lines should be fixed to the sides of the perfusion chamber with adhesive tape in such a way that a little tension is placed on the portal vein to simulate its normal tone. This also prevents the natural elasticity of the vessel pulling the venous cannula against the confluence of the portal and superior pancreatico-duodenal veins. Rhythmic contractions in the perfused portal vein are readily seen. A stitch should be placed in the duodenum and fixed to the perfusion chamber in a similar manner so that duodenal contractions do not disturb the pancreatic duct cannula. An appropriate graduated test-tube should be taped in position to collect pancreatic secretion. As has been previously described, the perfusion chamber is placed close by the water bath and the height adjusted so that a negative pressure of 2 to 3 cm of blood exists in the portal vein. Too high a negative venous pressure is not physiological and will suck the vein wall into the cannula and obstruct it. The preparation is washed with warmed Ringer's solution and checked for blood leaks. Blood loss should be negligible and certainly not exceed 0.5 ml/min. The preparation is covered with a polythene sheet and the perfusion chamber closed (Figure 69).

The temperature of the preparation should now be 37 or 38°C. The blood flow is increased until the venous oxygen saturation is about 65%. In practice, the blood flow is usually about 20 ml/min. The arterial oxygen saturation should be checked at the beginning of perfusion. Reference has already been made in Chapter 6 to the necessity for adding glucose to the blood in the perfusion circuit as well as sodium bicarbonate to maintain a normal pH and acid base relationship. Samples of venous blood should be taken at intervals. Should a reservoir be incorporated in the arterial line of the circuit, it is important to ensure that stagnation and separation of the blood does not occur. Arterial pressure is most simply monitored by connecting the cannula to a mercury manometer and making frequent

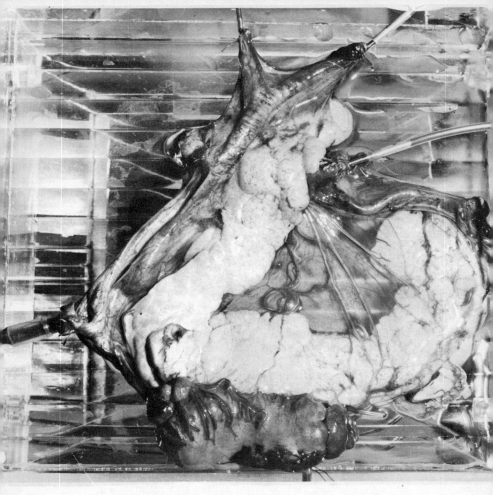

Fig. 69 Photograph of isolated perfused canine pancreas preparation. (The cover has been removed.) At the top of the frame arterial pressure, splenic arterial and superior mesenteric arterial cannulas are seen from left to right. Portal venous cannula on the left. Pancreatic duct cannula leaves via the duodenotomy at the extreme lower limit of the picture.

observations. It may, however, be connected via a transducer to an appropriate recorder. At the blood flow rate described, the arterial pressure at the beginning of perfusion usually lies between 80 and 110 mm Hg and indeed may rise in the first 15 minutes. Thereafter, a gradual fall in arterial pressure takes place over the subsequent 30–45 minutes to reach a level of about 30 mm Hg which then remains constant. This gradual decline does not, however, obscure the sharp drop in pressure that follows an injection of pure secretin, gastrin or cholecystokinin-pancreozymin into the arterial line. The flow of 95%

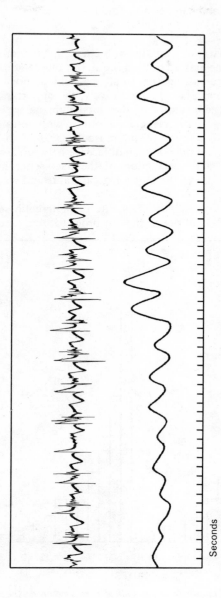

Seconds

Fig. 70 Simultaneous recordings of duodenal myoelectrical activity and intraluminal pressure in isolated perfused preparation. The frequency of the pacesetter potential is between 17 and 18 cycles per minute which is within normal limits for this part of the intestine. Action potentials are superimposed on the pacesetter potential and are associated with pressure changes in the duodenum.

oxygen and 5% carbon dioxide to the oxygenator should be as low as possible to minimise blood damage and fluid loss.

Function
As described, the preparation contains 4–6 cm of duodenum. Should the studies that are to be carried out require it, this duodenum may be separated from the pancreas, ligating small vessels, a manoeuvre that is tedious and often unnecessary. Alternatively, the opportunity may be taken to observe the reaction of the duodenum as well as the pancreas to a stimulus, monitoring its motility with intra-luminal balloons, the electrical activity of its muscular wall with serosal electrodes (Figure 70), and the potential difference between lumen and blood. The frequency and conduction of the pace-setter potential are a highly sensitive index of the physiological status and viability of the preparation.

Under basal conditions, a slow flow rate of pancreatic secretion continues at 0·05 to 0·1 ml per 5 min. In order to obtain sufficient

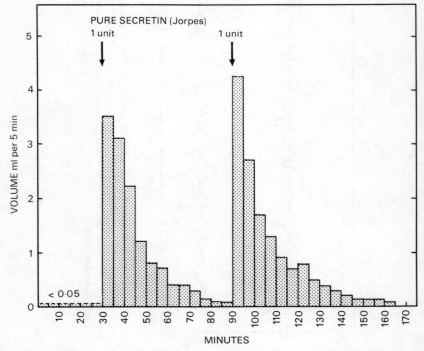

Fig. 71 Effect of repeated injections of one unit of pure secretin on the volume of pancreatic juice in the isolated perfused preparation.

material for enzyme and electrolyte determination it is often convenient to pool pancreatic secretion in 15-min samples. The research worker who, for the first time, establishes a successful perfusion, will be gratified to note that an injection of 1 unit of secretin into the arterial line is followed after a short interval by a brisk flow of clear watery secretion and a fall in arterial pressure (Figure 71). The anions and cations of the uncontaminated pancreatic secretion thus obtained may be measured, together with proteolytic enzymes – trypsinogen, chymotrypsinogen, procarboxypeptidase and others such as amylase, lipase and prophospholipase. The venous blood does, of course, issue directly from the pancreas, and proximal duodenum if this is included, and the levels of insulin and glucagon as well as the enzymes of the exocrine pancreas may be measured.

The isolated perfused canine pancreas may be studied for some hours whilst multiple functions are continuously observed. A considerable body of information may be obtained from tests using nanogram quantities of pure substances.

References

Babkin, B.P. and Starling, E.H. (1926) A method for the study of the perfused pancreas. *J. Physiol.* **61,** 245.

Delaney, J.P. and Custer, J. (1965) Gastrointestinal blood flow in the dog. *Circ. Res.* **17,** 394:

Nardi, G.L., Creep, J.M., Chambers, D.A., McCrae, C. and Skinner, D.B. (1963) Physiologic peregrinations in pancreatic perfusion. *Ann. Surg.* **158,** 830.

Hermon-Taylor, J. (1968) A technique for perfusion of the isolated canine pancreas: responses to secretin and gastrin. *Gastroenterology,* **55,** 488.

Perfusion of the Isolated Canine Gallbladder Duodenum and Pancreas

Introduction

Numerous *in vivo* (Vagne and Grossman, 1967, 1968; Ludwick and Bass, 1967; Higgins and Mann, 1926; Erspamer *et al,* 1967; Ivy and

Oldberg, 1928; Berry and Flower, 1971; Snape *et al*, 1948; Haver-mark and Hultman, 1953; Svatos *et al*, 1964, Hong *et al*, 1956; Pallin and Skoglund, 1964; Doyon, 1893) and *in vitro* studies (Mack and Todd, 1968; Berry and Flower, 1971; Agren, 1939; Hultman, 1954; Vane, 1964; Amer and Becvar, 1969) have been conducted on the motility of the gallbladder.

In man these have been limited mostly to radiological investigation of an opacified gallbladder (Lempke *et al*, 1963; Johnson and Boyden, 1952) and the influence of certain foods (Boyden, 1928), oral or intravenously administered drugs, or vagotomy (Johnson and Boyden, 1952) upon this. Obviously it is not possible to make direct measurements of pressure, or pressure changes within the normal human gallbladder.

In animals *in vivo* experiments (Vagne and Grossman, 1967, 1968; Ivy and Oldberg, 1928; Berry and Flower, 1971; Snape *et al*, 1948; Havermark and Hultman, 1952; Svatos *et al*, 1964; Hong *et al*, 1956; Pallin and Skoglund, 1964; Doyon, 1893) usually involve cannulation of this viscus by an incision in the fundus which may affect the function of the organ. *In vitro* studies (Mack and Todd, 1968; Berry and Flower, 1971; Agren, 1939; Hultman, 1954; Vane, 1964; Amer and Becvar, 1969) most commonly describe the response obtained in strips of gallbladder wall suspended in an organ bath to various pharmacological stimuli (Berry and Flower, 1971; Hultman, 1954).

As far as we know, no reports of studies carried out in the isolated perfused organ have been published. We have, however, had consider-able experience of the isolated perfused preparation of canine pan-creas and duodenum as previously described. It therefore seemed a logical extension to try and devise a method whereby the gallbladder could be included. Such a preparation would enable studies to be made which were free from the influence of certain hormonal or nervous factors which might operate in the intact animal.

Experiments were designed to investigate gallbladder motility and to study the effects of certain gastro-intestinal hormones on this.

To enable the gallbladder to be included in the preparation of pancreas, duodenum and upper jejunum, some modification is neces-sary in the arrangement of arterial perfusion and venous drainage used in the previous preparation.

Figure 72 shows the vascular connections used in this preparation. The main differences in the arterial supply are:

1. The hepatic artery and its branches to the gallbladder, common hepatic and common bile ducts, together with the cystic artery, are preserved and perfused. Only those branches of the hepatic artery

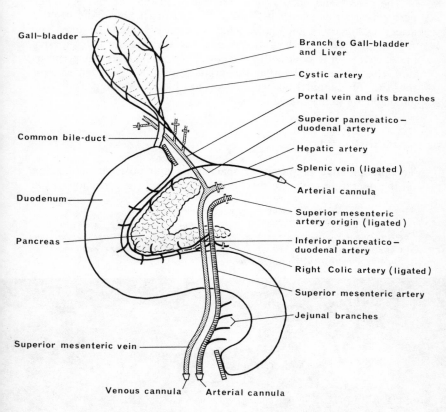

Gall–bladder

Common bile–duct

Duodenum

Pancreas

Superior mesenteric vein

Branch to Gall–bladder and Liver

Cystic artery

Portal vein and its branches

Superior pancreatico– duodenal artery

Hepatic artery

Splenic vein (ligated)

Arterial cannula

Superior mesenteric artery origin (ligated)

Inferior pancreatico– duodenal artery

Right Colic artery (ligated)

Superior mesenteric artery

Jejunal branches

Venous cannula   Arterial cannula

Fig. 72 Isolated perfused canine gallbladder. Vascular supply.

supplying the liver are ligated. This is in contrast to perfusion of the splenic artery in the previous preparation where the hepatic artery is ligated just beyond the origin of the superior pancreatico-duodenal artery. Perfusion of the hepatic artery not only simplifies the anatomical dissection but is necessary for an adequate blood supply to the gallbladder and extrahepatic bile duct system.

2. The superior mesenteric artery is again cannulated retrogradely but at a more distal level. This safeguards the arterial supply to distal duodenum, duodeno-jejunal flexure and proximal jejunum. The preservation of this added length of small bowel becomes important in experiments designed to demonstrate endogenous release of cholecystokinin from the bowel mucosa at this level (Berry and Flower, 1971).

The extent and adequacy of arterial perfusion can be seen after performing an arteriogram (Figure 73) and in particular the hepatic artery, cystic artery and choledochal anastomosis should be noted.

The difference in venous drainage is the use of the superior mesenteric vein in contrast to the portal vein in the previous preparation. Use of the portal vein in this preparation is not possible because the site of cannulation would prevent blood draining from the gallbladder and bile ducts.

Operative Procedure

The preoperative preparation, anaesthesia and position of the dog on the operating table are the same as described for perfusion of the

Fig. 73 Arteriogram of gallbladder preparation

1. *Hepatic Artery*
2. *Choledochal Anastomosis*
3. *Cystic Artery*
4. *Superior Pancreatico-Duodenal Artery*
5. *Superior Mesenteric Artery*
6. *Inferior PancreaticoèDuodenal Artery*
7. *Superior Mesenteric Vein*

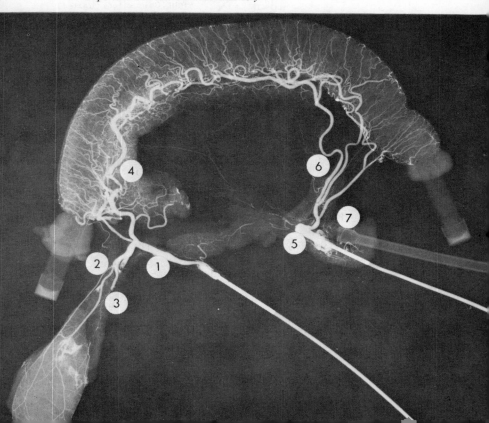

isolated pancreatic preparation. The perfusion apparatus (Figure 74) is similar to that described for the pancreas (Figure 65).

Preparation of Arterial and Venous Lines

The vessels in each groin are prepared for cannulation later in the experiment. The (R) femoral artery is used as a bleeding line to prime the circuit. The (R) femoral vein is employed to infuse 500 ml Krebs

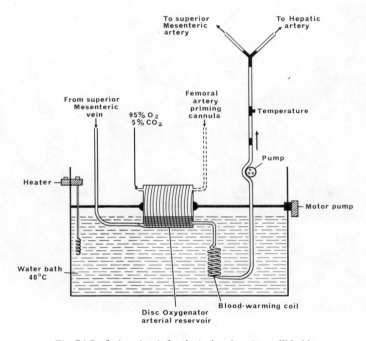

Fig. 74 Perfusion circuit for the isolated canine gallbladder.

solution during surgery which maintains an adequate state of hydration and helps to prevent the development of a metabolic acidosis. The femoral vein in the left groin is used to drain blood from the venous side of the circulation.

Initial Dissection, Preparation of Superior Mesenteric Vessels and of Distal End of Specimen

The abdomen is opened in the usual manner and good exposure, which is essential in the later part of the dissection, is maintained by stout hooks which distract the abdominal walls.

The duodenal ligament (Figure 75) is incised with diathermy as far over to the left side of the superior mesenteric artery as possible. The mesentery of the duodenum is then very gently separated from the superior mesenteric vessels by dissection in an avascular plane (Figure 76) – this is carried up as far as possible towards the origin of the superior mesenteric artery. Freeing this mesentery exposes the

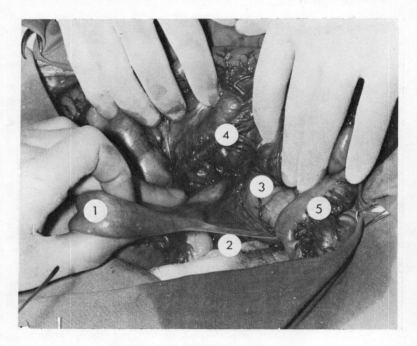

Fig. 75 Gallbladder preparation

1.	*Distal Duodenum*	*4.*	*Superior Mesenteric Vein*
2.	*Duodenal Ligament*	*5.*	*Ileum*
3.	*Colon*		

superior mesenteric vessels. Both artery and vein are prepared at this stage because tension can be applied to the undivided small bowel mesentery, which facilitates dissection of these vessels. If it is carried out after division of the colic, jejunal, and ileal branches tension is more difficult to apply to the stump and rotation also takes place which hinders a satisfactory technique.

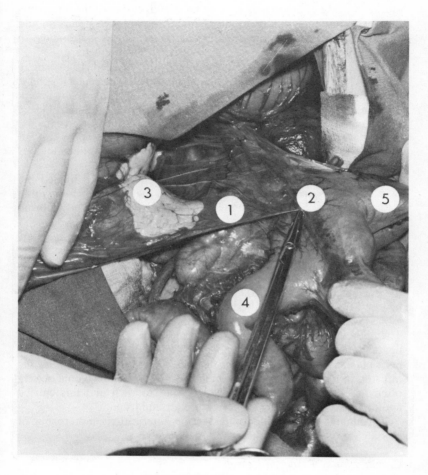

Fig. 76 Gallbladder preparation

1. Duodenal Mesentery	4. Terminal Ileum
2. Avascular Plane	5. Colon
3. Pancreas	

The visceral peritoneum covering the more distal part of these vessels should be diathermied before commencing dissection otherwise marked oozing of blood occurs from its cut edges due to the numerous fine vessels contained in the peritoneum at this site. Great care should be exercised in passing ligatures around these vessels as damage to venous tributaries can occur very easily during this manoeuvre.

The right colic vessels are next ligated and divided, followed by division of ileal and jejunal branches of the superior mesenteric artery, up to the selected level for division of duodenum or proximal jejunum. The small bowel is divided between double 30 thread ties, and before the proximal ligature is tied a wide-bore cannula is inserted into the bowel lumen and secured (Figure 77). This cannula provides an adequate means for escape of duodenal content or of solutions infused through the proximal end of the specimen.

The inferior mesenteric artery is next identified and divided between ligatures and stout ties placed around the upper rectum, which is then divided. Thus both small and large bowel are freed from all their attachments and are removed from the animal.

Preparation of Hepatic Arterial Line and Proximal End of Specimen

Attention is then turned towards the proximal end of the preparation. The gastro-splenic ligament is divided to display the vessels of the coeliac axis (Figure 78). The splenic and left gastric arteries are ligated in continuity and the hepatic artery (easily recognised by its looped course and surrounding nerve fibres) prepared for cannulation. The right gastric and right gastro-epiploic arteries are divided and ligated; the pylorus is next divided (Figure 79) and a similar large-bore plastic cannula inserted into the first part of the duodenum for infusion of desired solutions through this viscus. Troublesome oozing often takes place from the cut end of the stomach and this can be avoided by tying a further stout ligature around its end.

Throughout this period of dissection intermittent monitoring of blood gases is carried out using the Astrup method.

Cannulation of Prepared Vessels

The animal is heparinised with 7500 units of heparin, the first bleeding line is inserted into the right femoral artery and 200 ml of blood withdrawn to prime the apparatus and circuit. A further bleeding line is inserted into the right common carotid artery and clamped prior to bleeding the animal out, and its opposing vessel ligated in continuity. The left femoral artery is also ligated in continuity and via the left femoral vein a cannula is inserted into the I.V.C. as far up as the liver.

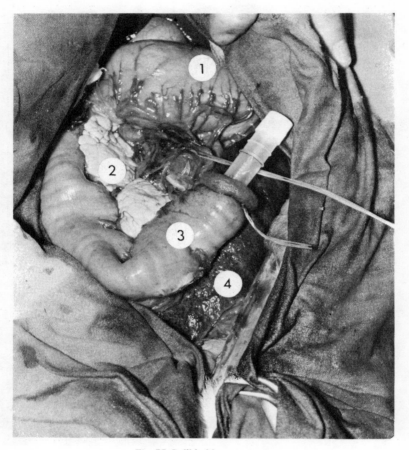

Fig. 77 Gallbladder preparation

1. *Stomach*
2. *Pancreas*
3. *Duodenum – Divided distal end with cannula inserted*
4. *Spleen*

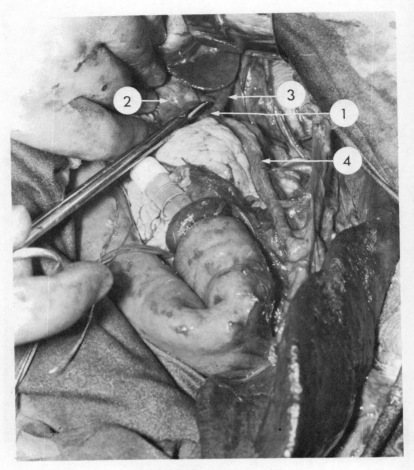

Fig. 78 Gallbladder preparation

1. Coeliac Axis
2. Hepatic Artery
3. (L) Gastric Artery
4. Splenic Artery

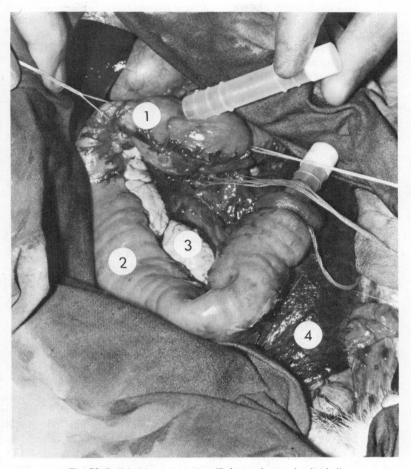

Fig. 79 Gallbladder preparation (Pylorus about to be divided)

1. Pylorus
2. Duodenum
3. Pancreas
4. Spleen

The next three manoeuvres are carried out as quickly as possible to avoid ischaemia of the preparation.

1. The superior mesenteric vein is cannulated.
2. The superior mesenteric artery is cannulated and as soon as the ligature has been tied the pump is switched on to commence perfusion.
3. The hepatic artery is cannulated and this line opened immediately for perfusion.

The animal is then bled out from

1. (R) femoral artery.
2. (R) common carotid artery
3. (L) femoral vein

The blood from 1. runs straight into the disc oxygenator (Figure 74), whilst from 2. and 3. it is collected into sterile bottles each containing 1000 units of heparin.

Isolation of the Vascular Supply

The superior mesenteric artery (at its origin from the aorta) and hepatic branches of the hepatic artery are clipped to prevent loss of blood into the general circulation, and a ligature tied around the inferior vena cava which contains the venous bleeding line.

The chest is then opened by dividing the sternum, as this greatly facilitates the dissection of the porta hepatis, and a ligature is placed around the suprahepatic segment of the I.V.C.

The final stages of isolation of the preparation are commenced by ligating and dividing the already clamped superior mesenteric artery close to its origin. The tissue on either side of this vessel is best ligated separately. The splenic vein is next secured and divided and attention is then turned to the branches of the portal vein and hepatic artery in the porta hepatis (Figure 80). On the (R) side there are usually 2 or 3 constant branches of both artery and vein and once their peritoneal coverings have been incised, a fully curved Stille forceps is used to dissect behind these vessels and pass ligatures around them. Once they have been divided mobilisation of the (R) side of the porta hepatis is complete. Similar dissection is carried out on the (L) side, followed by the superior aspect. It is not necessary to ligate the hepatic bile ducts at this stage.

Thus, all parts of the porta hepatis are now free except for the posterior aspect. It becomes a simple matter to lift this part of the preparation up to display the remaining branches (2–3 small vessels) which are then ligated and divided.

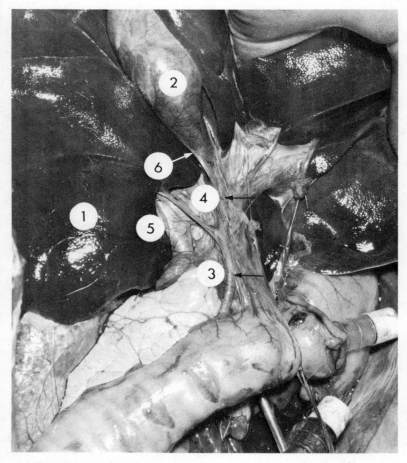

Fig. 80 Gallbladder preparation (liver reflected up to display porta hepatis).

1. Liver
2. Gallbladder
3. Common Bile Duct, with hepatic ducts draining into it above
4. Cystic Duct
5. Branch of Portal Vein
6. Cystic Artery

Dissection and Cannulation of the Gallbladder

Depending on the anatomy of the arterial supply to the gallbladder, great care must be taken not to ligate those branches of the hepatic artery which quite commonly supply the distal part of the body and fundus of this organ (Figure 81).

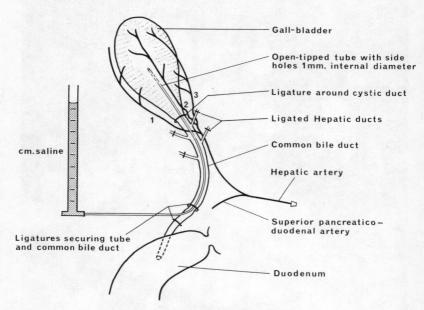

Fig. 81 Cannulation of gallbladder.

The gallbladder is then cannulated. A ligature is tied around the lower end of the common bile duct, a small opening is made in the duct, and a cannula (Portex 1·0 mm internal diameter O.T. with multiple side holes) passed up the duct and into the gallbladder. To ensure a closed system a ligature must be tied around the cystic duct, near its origin. If necessary, the cystic artery is dissected free from the cystic duct at this site so as not to be included in the tie. If this artery is included in the tie, then the main blood supply to the neck and proximal part of the body of the gallbladder is compromised.

The preparation now remains attached only by adherence of the gallbladder to the liver. Diathermy is used to complete this excision and it has been found best to leave a collar of liver tissue attached around the gallbladder. Troublesome bleeding otherwise takes place from numerous fine vessels on this aspect of the organ, which it is difficult to stop without damaging its wall. Any larger bleeding vessels in the collar of attached liver tissue are coagulated with diathermy.

Removal of Preparation from Dog to Perfusion Box

This is best done with both hands, and not instruments, as less damage is likely to occur. The arterial and venous lines must be held in their correct position otherwise they are liable to undergo twisting with resultant ischaemia on the arterial side, or venous congestion of the preparation if the superior mesenteric vein is involved.

The preparation is placed in the perfusion box and the lines secured in a satisfactory position. The gallbladder cannula is connected via a transducer and amplifier to a direct recording apparatus for pressure measurements.

Assessment of the Preparation

Absolute assessment of the isolated perfused gallbladder preparation can only be made by comparison with the effects of known pharmacological and physiological stimuli in the intact animal. The results of *in vitro* experiments may also be used as a parameter for comparative study.

However, various other methods of assessment have been used in this preparation. These include:

1. The macroscopic appearance of the preparation both initially and at the end of perfusion – a period of about three hours.

2. The histological appearance both initially and after three hours' perfusion.

3. The ability of the gallbladder to respond satisfactorily throughout the period of perfusion, together with continued motility of the duodenal segment.

4. The demonstration of an adequate arterial supply. This may be seen in Figure 73, an arteriogram of the vascular anatomy in this preparation.

5. Finally, comparison may be made between the pancreatic and duodenal activity responses obtained in this preparation and in the isolated preparation of pancreas and duodenum only.

Studies Which May be Carried Out

1. Measurement of resting gallbladder pressure.
2. Response of the gallbladder to various drugs and in particular to

gastro-intestinal hormones – this provides an assessment not only of isolated gallbladder activity, but of the comparative cholecystokinetic potencies of the individual hormones.

Figure 82 demonstrates the response of the gallbladder to cholecystokinin (3·2 Ivy dog units) injected into the arterial line. There was a short latent period followed by a sharp rise in gallbladder pressure which was sustained over the next 40 minutes. Below are the blood pressure and duodenal activity traces.

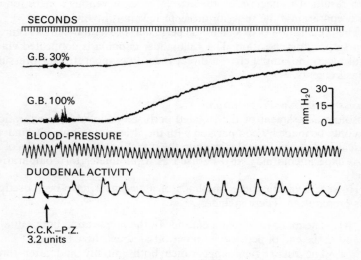

Fig. 82 Isolated gallbladder preparation.
Record of trace of resting preparation to injection of cholecystokinin into arterial line.

3.   Stimulation of the divided distal end of the hepatic nerve plexus and the observation of its effect on the gallbladder.

4.   More recently work has been carried out to try to demonstrate endogenous release of a substance from the duodenum which will contract the gallbladder. We have found that following perfusion of the duodenum with a solution of proteoses and peptones an increase in intracholecystic pressure can be obtained. However, a considerable amount of further work needs to be carried out before any definite conclusions are reached concerning this study.

References

Agren, G. (1939) Preparation of cholecystokinin. *Scand. Arch. Physiol.* **81,** 234.

Amer, M.S., and Becvar, V.E. (1969) A sensitive *in vitro* method for the assay of cholecystokinin. *J. Endocr.* **43,** 637.

Berry, H., and Flower, R.J. (1971) The assay of endogenous cholecystokinin and factors influencing its release in the dog and cat. *Gastroenterology,* **60,** 409.

Boyden, E.A. (1928) An analysis of the reaction of the human gallbladder to food. *Anat. Rec.* **40,** 147.

Doyon, M. (1893) Contribution à l'étude de la contractilité des voies biliaires. Application de la méthode graphique à cette étude. *Arch. Physiol. Norm. Path.* **5,** 678.

Erspamer, V., Bertaccini, G., De Caro, G., Endean, R., and Impicciatore, M. (1967) Pharmacological actions of caerulein. *Experientia.* **23,** 702.

Havermark, P.G. and Hultman, E.H. (1952) A method of recording the contraction of the gallbladder *in situ,* its application to cholecystokinin determination. *Acta Physiol. Scand.* **27,** 242.

Higgins, G.M. and Mann, F.C. (1926) Emptying of the gallbladder, *Amer. J. Physiol.* **78,** 339.

Hong, S.S., Magee, D.G., and Crewdson, F. (1956) The physiologic regulation of gallbladder evacuation. *Gastroenterology.* **30,** 625.

Hultman, E.H. (1954) A method for the standardization of cholecystokinin *in vitro. Acta. Physiol. Scand.* **33,** 291.

Ivy, A.C., and Oldberg, E. (1928) A hormone mechanism for gallbladder contraction and evacuation. *Amer. J. Physiol.* **86,** 599.

Johnson, F.E., and Boyden, E.A. (1952) The effect of double vagotomy on the motor activity of the human gallbladder. *Surgery.* **32,** 591.

Lempke, R.E., King, R.D., and Kaiser, G.C. (1963) Hydrodynamics of gallbladder filling. *J. Amer. Med. Ass.* **186,** 152.

Ludwick, J.R. and Bass, P. (1967) Contractile and electric activity of the extrahepatic biliary tract and duodenum. *Surg. Gynec. Obstet.* **124,** 536.

Mack, A.J. and Todd, J.K. (1968) A study of human gallbladder *in vitro. Scot. Med. J.* **13,** 97.

Pallin, B., and Skoglund, S. (1964) Neural and humoral control of the gallbladder emptying mechanism in the cat. *Acta. Physiol. Scand.* **60,** 358.

Snape, W.J., Freidman, M.H.F., and Thomas, J.E. (1948) The assay of cholecystokinin and the influence of vagotomy on the gallbladder response. *Gastroenterology.* **10,** 496.

Svatos, A., Bartos, V.L. and Brzeck, V. (1964) Concentration of cholecystokinin in human lymph and serum. *Arch. Int. Pharmacodyn.* **149,** 515.

Vane, J.R. (1964) The use of isolated organs for detecting active substances in the circulating blood. *Brit. J. Pharmacol.* **23,** 360.

Vagne, M. and Grossman, M.I. (1968) Cholecystokinetic potency of gastro-intestinal hormones and related peptides. *Amer. J. Physiol.* **215,** (4) 881.

Vagne, M. and Grossman, M.I. (1967) Effect of gastrin on motility of gallbladder. *The Physiologist.* **10,** 330.

Index

Acid secretion 159, 160
  failure 135, 136, 158
Acidosis 141
Airway 24
  in the pig 27
Althesin 22
Ammonia 89, 91
Anaesthesia 20–29, 71
  adverse effects 20
  and the isolated liver 100–111
  by inhalation 20, 112
  by intraperitoneal injection 22, 128
  by intravenous injection 20, 21, 22, 76, 144
  for canine liver preparation 76
  for gallbladder preparation 194
  for pancreatic preparation 180
  for porcine liver preparation 112
  for rat liver preparation 128
  for stomach preparation 144
  inadequate 24
  maintenance 20, 23–24
Anaesthetic techniques
  dog 26
  pig 27
  rat 26
Anastomosis, choledochal 194
Angiography 58
Animal, choice of 16–19, 145
Anoxia 136, 142
Anti-foam 42

toxic effects 43
Aorta
  cannulation 147
  dissection 146, 148, 149
Apparatus 30–51
  bacterial infection 50
  cleaning 48, 126
  disposable 12
Arterial PCO$_2$ 24, 26
Arterial pressure 52, 57, 82
Arteries of the dog
  carotid, common 144, 145, 147, 198, 202
  coeliac axis 142, 143, 145, 146, 147, 173, 182, 198, 200
  colic 193, 198
  cystic 192, 193, 194, 203, 204
  femoral 76, 145, 147, 180, 195, 198, 202
  gastric 143, 173, 182, 198, 200
  gastro-epiploic (R) 182, 198
  hepatic 57, 76, 77, 79, 116, 142, 173, 186, 192, 193, 194, 198, 200, 202
  inferior mesenteric 146, 185
  lumbar 146, 148
  pancreatico-duodenal inferior 142, 143, 173–174, 183, 185, 193, 194, 198
  pancreatico-duodenal superior 173–174, 193, 194

renal   146–147
splenic   142, 146, 173–174, 180,
    182, 186, 193, 198, 200
superior mesenteric   78, 142, 143,
    145, 146–147, 173, 180, 183–185,
    186, 193, 194, 195, 198, 202
Arteries of the pig
    hepatic   112, 113, 114
Arteries of the rat
    hepatic   121
Arteriogram
    gallbladder   194
    pancreas   175
    stomach   143
Assessment of preparations
    canine liver   87
    gallbladder   205
    pancreas   190
    rat liver   130
    stomach   150, 151
Automatic mechanical ventilator   21

Baboon   72
Bicarbonate   83, 84, 92
Bile   57
    clearance studies   88, 89
    common bile duct   77, 88
    composition   88
    flow   73, 88, 114–120
    from isolated perfused canine liver
        116, 117, 118, 119
    from isolated perfused porcine liver
        114
Bile ducts
    common   193, 202, 204
    cystic   203, 204
    hepatic   203
Biliary obstruction   92
    anaesthetic agents in   105–106, 107
Bilirubin   88, 92
Biochemical parameters   151, 152
Biopsy, liver   79, 90, 94
Block, hepatic venous outflow   71–74,
    84
Blood damage
    by oxygenators   41
    by pumps   32
Blood flow   61
    monitoring   33
    non-pulsatile   34
    pulsatile   34
Blood gas tensions   42, 64

Blood pressure   61–62
Boyle's anaesthetic machine   20
Bromosulphthalein   88
    bypass, cardiopulmonary   71, 72

Caerulein, effect on porcine liver   116
Calf   17, 72
Cannulae
    choice of   45–46, 47
    in canine liver preparation   77, 78,
        79
    in gallbladder preparation   193, 198,
        202, 204–205
    in pancreas preparation   180, 185–
        187
    in porcine liver preparation   113
    in rat liver preparation   125
Cat   16, 72
Catecholamines   10, 140
    release during bleeding   10
Cavitation   9
Cholate excretion from porcine liver
    116
Chromium[51]   90
Circuit, perfusion. See Perfusion circuit
Citrate   53
Cleaning of apparatus   48–50, 126
    bacterial infection   50
Cross circulation   159
Cruelty to Animals Act (1876)   24
    non-depolarising muscle relaxants and
        24, 106
    suxamethonium and   24, 106

Dextran   55
Diaphragm   79, 80
Dirofilaria immitis   86
Disc oxygenator   39, 138, 195
Disposable apparatus   12
Dog
    advantages of the greyhound   17, 52
    anaesthesia and the isolated liver
        100–110
    gallbladder preparation   191–208
    liver preparation   71–100
    pancreas preparation   171–191
    stomach preparation   135–170
Duodenum   77, 146-
    dissection   195, 198
    ligament   196
    mesentery   197

Electrical activity 151–156, 165–168
  duodenum and pancreas 190
  gastro-oesophageal sphincter 165
  methodology 153
  stomach 153–155, 157
Electrodes 150, 154, 165, 190
Electrolytes 52, 54, 65, 92
  bicarbonate 65
  calcium 66
  potassium 65
  sodium and chloride 65
Elevated succinate levels 110
Endotoxin 84
Endotracheal tubes 21
Experimental team and their duties 12

Feasibility of organ perfusion 2
Fibrinogen 52
Flow
  gravity feed 56, 73
  portal 78, 79, 131
  rate 56–58, 73, 84, 93
  total hepatic 56
Flow meter, electromagnetic 61
Fluid, perfusion. See Perfusion fluid
Future of isolated organ perfusion 3

Gallbladder
  anatomy 193, 194
  arterial supply 193, 194, 202
  cannulation and dissection 204
  cannulation of vessels 198, 202
  isolation of vessels 202
  operative procedure 194–205
  pre-operative preparation 194
  preparation of arterial and venous
    lines 195–198
  recording of activity 206
  studies on, in vitro and in vivo 192
Gas mixtures 41, 42
Gas tensions 42
Gastro-oesophageal junction, trans-
    mucosal potential difference
    changes 161
Gastro-oesophageal sphincter 161
  electrical activity 165
  length 162
  pressure 162
  response to oesophageal distension
    163
Glucose 66, 73, 92, 151, 152
Goat 17, 72

Haematocrit 52, 63, 73, 75, 83, 87
Haemoglobin, free 53
Haemolysis 53, 62, 144
Heat exchangers 32, 137
Heparin 54, 71, 75, 78, 86, 113, 141,
    147, 198, 202
Hormones
  cholecystokinin 193, 205
  endogenous release of 193, 205
Humidity 62
Hypothermia 88
Hypoxia 24, 110
  in perfused organs 10

Induction of anaesthesia 21
Inhalation of volatile agents 23
  cyclopropane 23
  diethyl ether 23
  halothane 23, 110
Initial preparation for anaesthesia 21
  atropine 21
  premedication 21
Innulin space 20
Intubation in the pig 27

Ketamine 23
Krebs solution 54, 75, 77

Lactate clearance 89
Lactate/pyruvate ratio 89, 110
Ligament
  duodenal 196
  gastrosplenic 198
Liver
  advantages of the canine 100
  anaesthetic for 76, 112
  bile flow from 73, 88, 114–120
  B.S.P. secretion 114
  choice of type of perfusion 132
  circuit 74–76, 111–112, 122–125
  effects of anaesthetic agents 100–
    110
  failure 73
  isolated perfused canine 71–100
  isolated perfused porcine 111–120
  isolated perfused rat 120–134
  operative procedure 76–82,
    112–114, 128–129
  P.C.V. in 82, 114
  total tissue water 90
  transplantation 72
  weight 79, 83, 93

Low blood flow   110
Lowered oxygen tension   110
Lymph
    flow   90–92
    hepatic   57, 84
Lymphatics, hepatic   81, 82

Malayan pit viper venom   53
Malignant hypothermia in the pig   27
Metabolic acidosis   64
Metabolism   104–105
    biliary excretion   105
Microthrombi   53
Monitoring   60–67, 82–87
Monitoring during anaesthesia   25–26
    acid-base changes   25
    arterial pressure   25
    body temperature   25
    central venous pressure   (CVP)   25
Motility   156
    duodenal   158
    gastric   158
    small bowel   56
Muscle relaxants   24–25, 106
    alcuronium   106
    ^{14}C-pancuronium   106
    ^{14}C-tubocurarine   106
    gallamine   106
    histamine release   106
    metabolism and excretion in the
        bile   106
    pancuronium   106
    suxamethonium   106

Nitrous oxide   20, 24

Obstruction
    biliary   92
    hepatic venous   71–74, 84
Oedema   10, 54–55, 57, 88, 90
Oesophagus, dissection   149
Operative procedure
    gallbladder   194–205
    liver   76–82, 112–114, 128–129
    pancreas   180–187
    stomach   144–150
Organ chamber   31, 33, 138
Oxygen   20
    saturation   56, 73, 83, 84, 139
    uptake   56, 87
Oxygenator   31, 39
    Aga   73, 74

bubble   40, 86
disc   40
hooker   72
membrane   41
roller   41

Pancreas   56, 77, 78, 146, 171–191
    ampulla   177
    anatomy   173
    arterial supply   173–4
    blood flow   173, 187, 188
    ducts   176, 178
    duodenum   189, 190
    function of   190–191
    isolated perfusion of   171
    operative design   180
    operative procedure   180–187
    perfusion apparatus   177
    venous drainage   174
PCO_2 83
Pentagastrin
    effect on canine bile   116, 117
    effect on porcine bile   114, 115, 116
Perfusion circuit
    canine liver   74–76
    gallbladder   195
    pancreas   177–179
    porcine liver   111
    rat liver   122–125
    stomach   137–141
Perfusion fluid   52–55
    anticoagulation   53, 54, 75, 86
    blood autologous   52, 72, 86
    choice of   25, 75, 114, 126–128
    electrolytes   54
    haematocrit   52, 73, 75
    protein   52, 54, 55, 75, 94
Perfusion of organs
    basic requirements and principles   9
    combination of organs   3
    deterioration in preparation   13
    experimental procedure   13
    extent of perfusion   12
    prolonged experiments   4
Perfusion pressure   61
    measurement of   64
Ph   63–64, 83, 84, 87
    arterial   64
    arterio-venous reversal   64
    perfusion values   64
    physiological range   64
    venous   64

Phosphatase, alkaline   88, 92
Pig   72, 111–120
   advantages of   17
Plasma proteins   66
Plasminogen   53
PO$_2$ 64
Polyvinylchloride   43
   toxicity of   44
Porcine liver
   isolated perfused   111–120
Porta hepatis   202, 203
Potassium   73, 92
Pressure
   arterial   52, 57, 82
   hepatic venous   79, 82–84
   osmotic   52
   portal venous   57, 73, 82, 125, 131
   venous, in perfused stomach   137
Priming volume   9
   use of autologous blood   10
Pulse pressure   39
   and tissue damage   39
Pumps   32, 33
   Dale-Schuster   72
   non-pulsatile   33, 34
   pulsatile   33, 36, 37, 38
   roller   35, 37
   roller-occlusive   74
   screw type   74
Pylorus, pressure profile   159

Rat   16, 72
Rat liver perfusion   120–134
   advantages   120
   apparatus   30
   ATP   132
   cannulae   125
   choice of perfusion   131
   cleaning of apparatus   126
   constant flow   122
   constant pressure   129
   criteria of satisfactory perfusion   130
   disadvantages   122
   effect of erythrocytes   132
   filters   125
   gluconeogenesis   121, 127, 131
   operative techniques   128
   oxygenator   124
   perfusion media   126–128
   Ph control   124
   portal pressure   125, 131

   tubing   126
Reservoirs   74
   venous   48, 49

Secretin
   effect on canine bile   116, 118
   effect on porcine bile   114–116
Shunts, arteriovenous   57, 58
Slow waves
   abnormality   156
   duodenum   153, 157
   propagation   153, 157
   site of origin   156, 157
   stomach   153, 155, 157
Sodium taurocholate
   effect on canine bile   116, 119
   effect on porcine bile   114, 115, 116
Stomach   56, 77, 135–170
   acid secretion   135–136, 159–161
   arterial supply   142
   electrical activity   153–158
   motility   158, 159
   operative procedure   144–150

Tachygastria   156
Temperature   25, 73, 74, 83
Temperature regulation   31, 32
Thermocouple   75, 83
Thiopentone sodium   22
Tissue compartment size   90
Transmucosal potential difference   163
Transplantation, liver   72
Tubing   43–45, 71, 74, 86, 126
   PVC toxicity test   45

Urea   92, 94

Vapouriser   21
Veins of the dog
   femoral   78, 145, 186, 195, 198, 202
   inferior vena cava   74, 76, 78, 137,
      144, 147, 202
   pancreatico-duodenal   77, 143, 145,
      146, 147, 174, 176, 185, 187
   portal   73, 76, 143–144, 145, 147,
      176, 180, 186–187, 193, 194, 202
   splenic   77, 143, 148, 173, 174, 193,
      202
   superior mesenteric   78, 143–144,
      145, 146, 147, 174, 183, 193, 194,
      196, 202

Veins of the pig
   femoral   112
   inferior vena cava   111, 113
   portal   112, 113, 114
Veins of the rat
   inferior vena cava   125, 128
   portal   121, 125, 128
Venous drainage   143, 194
Venous obstruction   139
Ventilation   20
Viscosity   53, 83
Volatile anaesthetic agents and the isolated canine liver   101

chloroform   101
enzyme activity   101
glucose and potassium balance   101
halothane   101
^{14}C-halothane   104, 105
methoxyflurane   101

Water, bath   75

Xenon^{133} 57
   blood flow measurement   62, 160